DIABETES EPIDEMIC & YOU

Should Everyone Be Tested?

ABSOLUTELY NOT!
ONLY
THOSE CONCERNED ABOUT THEIR FUTURE!

Joseph R. Kraft, MD, MS, FCAP

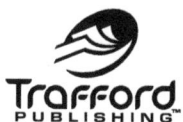

Order this book online at www.trafford.com
or email orders@trafford.com

Most Trafford titles are also available at major online book retailers.

© Copyright 2008, 2011 Joseph R. Kraft, MD.
All rights reserved. No part of this publication may be reproduced, stored in a retrieval system, or transmitted, in any form or by any means, electronic, mechanical, photocopying, recording, or otherwise, without the written prior permission of the author.

Note for Librarians: A cataloguing record for this book is available from Library and Archives Canada at www.collectionscanada.ca/amicus/index-e.html

Printed in the United States of America.

ISBN: 978-1-4251-6809-4 (sc)
ISBN: 978-1-4251-7812-3 (hc)
ISBN: 978-1-4251-6811-7 (e)

Trafford rev. 03/02/2011

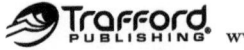 www.trafford.com

North America & international
toll-free: 1 888 232 4444 (USA & Canada)
phone: 250 383 6864 ♦ fax: 812 355 4082

Joseph R. Kraft, MD, MS, FCAP

Diplomate

American Board of Pathology
Anatomic pathology   Clinical pathology

Diplomate

American Board of Nuclear Medicine

Chairman Emeritus

Department of Clinical Pathology
And Nuclear Medicine

St. Joseph Hospital
Chicago, IL USA

To Mary Catherine, the love of my life

To our family

Adrienne, Cheryl, Gregory, Stephen, Kevin, Mark, Joan, Michele, and Regina

To our grandchildren

Kristen, Brian, Darren, Timothy, Raymond,

Nicholas, Christopher, Nicole, Alexandra, Anna, Chloe and Conrad

To our great-grandchildren

Braiden, Taylor, and Kathryn Nicole

For whom it is hoped that the Diabetes Epidemic will be conquered soon.

Preface-2011

Diabetes Epidemic and You

The subsequent book reviews were received following the first printing in 2008.

※※

Diabetes Epidemic and You is superbly written, in a language that is accessible to the general public and yet precise enough for physicians. It is a difficult thing to achieve such clarity. Besides, it is a complete book that includes all related subjects in perfect manner.

Prof. Dr. Pedro Luiz Mangabeira Albernaz
Professor of Otorhinolaryngology
Escola Paulista de Medicina
Universidade Federal de Sao Paulo
Sao Paulo, Brasil

*　　*　　*　　*　　*　　*　　*　　*　　*　　*　　*

The International Tinnitus Journal Volume 15, Number 1, 2009

Joseph Kraft has written a book entitled *Diabetes Epidemic and You*. The subtitle is even more important and timely: *Should Everyone Be Tested? Absolutely Not! Only Those Concerned About Their Future!* In this very speedily readable book, Dr. Kraft outlines the history of diabetes and the discovery of insulin and its assays. He then goes on to relate his experience with 14,384 assays from 1972 through 1998. From there, the author puts together the relationship of insulin levels, blood sugar, and diabetes.

To complete the book, the second part compiles the age distribution of these oral glucose tolerances with insulin assays. This comparison not so subtly reveals the importance of this testing from age 3 to 90+ years.

This wonderful written book is suitable both for the public and for the profession. It is a treasure of knowledge and experience not otherwise available. This work should be required reading for all medical students, endocrinologists, otolaryngologists, and anybody interested in their future – and especially for physicians concerned about their future and that of their patients.

Kenneth H. Brookler, MD, MS, FRCSC
Clinical Professor of Otolaryngology
New York Medical College
Valhalia, New York

The International Tinnitus Journal Volume 15, Number 1 2009

This is a wonderful text both for the public and for our profession because of the tremendous amount of knowledge that reflects what we do know and what can occur later. There is no question that the body's biochemistry and neural mechanisms rely on our intake of food or exposure to other chemicals. Therefore, as diabetes affects these entities, they also affect our body in relation to all other illnesses.

This is a superb textbook that should be read by the public, by members of our profession while in training, and those who are in practice so that they will begin to understand and expect what is occurring biochemically. It is a book for the present and for the future, and it deserves great commendations.

Wallace Rubin, M.D.
Clinical Professor, Department of Otolaryngology
Louisiana State University School of Medicine
New Orleans, LA

"The goal of this book is to awaken the silent millions with undiagnosed diabetes to combat the Diabetes epidemic beginning with you - and I do mean you." states the author, Joseph R. Kraft, MD, chairman of the Department of Clinical Pathology and Nuclear Medicine, St. Joseph Hospital, Chicago, Illinois, 1962-1998.

In a comprehensive, well planned manner, the book integrates and provides to the medical community, clinicians, research professionals, and patients an extensive autopsy and clinical pathology experience for a practical approach to the diagnosis, treatment, and control of the pathogenesis of type 2 diabetes. "The earliest diagnosis of prediabetes is hyperinsulin, type 2 diabetes, identified by the oral glucose tolerance test with insulin assay with normal glucose tolerance."

Since 1921, the oral glucose tolerance test has been an established procedure for the early diagnosis of diabetes. The focus of the reported clinical experience in this book is the application since 1972 at St. Joseph's Hospital of the oral glucose tolerance test with insulin assays for the early diagnosis of diabetes. "This test has provided the earliest diagnosis of prediabetes and diabetes even when the blood sugars were normal."

Diabetes Epidemic and You / JOSEPH R. KRAFT MD

Dr. Kraft's book is recommended as a source of information to professionals and patients of all ages interested in the maintenance of good health. All join with the author in attempting to influence and limit the clinical progression of the "diabetes epidemic." This volume is a step forward for achieving the author's ultimate goal: "the prevention of the pathology of diabetes mellitus and cardiovascular disease."

Abraham Shulman, M.D., FACS
Professor Emeritus Clinical Otolaryngology
State University of New York
Health Science Center at Brooklyn, New York

The earliest identification of diabetes persists as an enigma and a persistent challenge to international clinical medicine. William Osler, M.D., in his classic text, *The Principles and Practice of Medicine (1892)* was unable to identify a beginning of diabetes other than hyperglycemia. However, he noted age differences. Diabetes beginning in children, all of whom had a short survival and diabetes beginning in adulthood, had much in common. There were no cures and no ultimate survival.

In adult diabetes, Osler noted frequent urination as an early sign of diabetes. The urine did not always contain sugar. Occasionally, diabetes insipidus was identified. Unknown at that time was that arteriosclerosis of the kidneys could elevate the renal threshold for sugar thereby resulting in negative urines.

Doctor Osler, a distinguished Professor of Medicine, John Hopkins University, was fully aware that the autopsy was a pillar of medicine. He personally performed many autopsies. His pathology dissertations were extensive, especially on arteriosclerosis equal to that of today. Dr. Osler was a physician, a clinician, and truly a clinical pathologist.

During Osler's time, arteriosclerosis was treated as an independent affection of the vascular system being an involution process accompanying old age as an expression of the natural wear and tear of the vessels. Longevity according to Osler was a vascular question. He so well expressed this in the axiom – "a man is only as old as his arteries." To a majority of men, death came primarily or secondarily through this portal just as it does today.

When arteriosclerosis occurred in the young, he attributes it to an inherited event. Osler noted that – "a man of twenty-eight or twenty-nine may have {the} arteries of sixty {year old} and a man of forty may present vessels as much degenerated as should be at eighty." (*See Chapter 14. Pathology of Type 1 Diabetes.*) The concept that arteriosclerosis, heart failure, and diabetes, are simply an aging event, as expressed by Osler prevails today. Unfortunately, it remains a cornerstone of the "silent" diabetes epidemic today.

Dr. Osler was ahead of his time. The following events are highlighted:

1890 – Minkowski and Von Mering's discovery that dogs developed severe diabetes immediately after pancreatectomy. This stimulated the idea of treating diabetes with pancreatic tissue.

1892 – The Principles and Practice of Medicine, New York, D. Appleton and Company, 1892 Osler cited that sub-total pancreatectomy did not produce diabetes.

1893 – Edward Laguesse suggested that the clump of cells described by Dr. Langerhans in his doctorate thesis (1869) be named the Islets of Langerhans and that they might constitute the endocrine tissue of the pancreas.

1909 – Dr. Jean de Meyer gave the name "insulin" to the glucose lowering hormone when its existence was still hypothetical.

1918 – Janney and Isaacson initiated the 100-g 3-h sugar tolerance intended to evaluate and diagnosis endocrine disorders and only secondary for diabetes.

1922 – Insulin discovered; Banting and Macleod received Nobel Prize (1923).

1925 – The oral glucose tolerance 100-g 3-h procedure was standardized and considered of great value in the early diagnosis of prediabetes and diabetes. (See Chapter 13.)

1975 – Detection of diabetes mellitus in-situ (occult diabetes). (See Chapter 12.)

The very earliest diagnosis of diabetes identified hyperinsulinemia by insulin assay with normal glucose tolerance occurred in 1975. Dr. Stout's investigations and research of the 1970's identified increased insulin (hyperinsulinemia) as a primary cause affecting all arterial vessels including capillaries. This accounted for the microangiopathy of the retina, the neurotology of the central and peripheral nervous system and the arteriosclerosis of all major and minor arteries. The latter was so aptly described by Dr. Osler in his 1892 text.

The very earliest diagnosis of diabetes is neither by fasting blood sugars nor by glycated hemoglobin but only by insulin assays with normal glucose tolerance as affirmed in this text. This resource of 14,384 oral glucose tolerance with insulin assay is unequaled in world medical publications. (*See Chapter 14 – Pathology of Type 2 Diabetes.*)

It must also be noted that type 1 diabetics, all of whom received exogenous (long-acting) insulin over their lifetime are thereby made hyperinsulinemic. As a consequence, the pathology of type 1 diabetes is now indistinguishable from the hyperinsulin (insulin resistant) pathology of type 2 diabetes, beginning with cardiovascular disease.

Cholesterol: Friend or Foe?

Cholesterol is a fat-like substance in all of our body cells including blood. Our bodies need cholesterol. It is essential for our very existence. Without it, we are no more. It consists of a low-density lipoprotein (LDL) and a high density lipoprotein component. An anatomic pathology for cholesterol does not exist. A pathologic relationship of cholesterol per se to arteriosclerosis is lacking. Cholesterol among several lipids is a co-participant in lipid deposition in arterial vessels damaged by hyperinsulinemia (insulin resistance) in the production of athero-arteriosclerosis. (*See Chapter 19.*)

STOP DIABETES

The Professional Section Quarterly Fall 2009, News from the American Diabetes Association cited *"New Campaign to Stop Diabetes has been launched."* According to survey results released in November 2009 by the ADA, Americans earned a score of 51% when asked a series of questions about a disease so common that it strikes every 20 seconds. To raise awareness of diabetes and its consequences, the ADA launched the new movement, *"STOP DIABETES".* The Association campaign aims to put a halt to this lack of awareness and misinformation, so the direction of prevalence in this country can change.

Until the earliest diagnosis of type 2 diabetes, which is the insulin assay with normal glucose tolerance is utilized, the *"STOP DIABETES"* campaign, a most needed program, will be incomplete.

In the absence of personal exposure to autopsy pathology of type 2 diabetes, clinicians and clinical investigators, including those from distinguished institutions, continue to fail to connect the pathology of diabetes with the earliest diagnosis of diabetes and its clinical pathogenesis, e.g. athero-arteriosclerosis.

Since 1970, the autopsy – with the exception of forensic requirements – has virtually become obsolete to the detriment of clinical medicine. Hence, graduates in medicine from 1970 on, through no fault of their own, have been deprived of this continuum of autopsy knowledge. Magnetic Resonance Imaging (MRI) and other modalities yet to be are not substitutes for the autopsy, which remains the pillar of medicine, as it was in the time of Osler.

Cardiovascular disease conferences are legion. They excel in addressing clinical management and life saving advances. The conferences, irrespective of sponsorship and faculty, fail to address the hyperinsulinemia, (insulin resistant) pathogenesis of arteriosclerosis. In this relative absence of significant autopsy experience or exposure, the conferences reflect a collective lack of understanding of the vascular autopsy pathology of type 1 and type 2 diabetes. The type 1 diabetic by receiving exogenous insulin over their lifetime becomes hyperinsulinemic (insulin resistant). The pathology of type 1 diabetes is now indistinguishable from hyperinsulinemic (insulin resistant) pathology of type 2 diabetes. (*See Chapter 14.*)

Cardiovascular conferences designate cardiovascular disease as a risk factor for diabetes. The predominate pathologies of hyperinsulinemia, type 2 diabetes are athero-arteriosclerosis, cardiovascular disease, cerebral vascular disease, hypertension, nephropathy, retinopathy, peripheral and central neuropathy, and penile erectile dysfunction. They have their beginning when the blood sugars are normal. (*See Chapter 14.*) **The pathologies of diabetes are not risk factors for diabetes. They are the clinical pathology of diabetes! If you have any of the pathologies of diabetes, you are diabetic irrespective of your glucose status!**

In the undiagnosed with any of the clinical pathologies noted above, especially those with normal fasting blood sugars, the insulin assay with oral glucose tolerance will confirm the diabetes diagnosis.

Insulin deficiency (hypoinsulinemia) is the prima facie of type 1 diabetes. Direct measurements of insulin determining normal, increased (hyperinsulin) and decreased (hypoinsulin) have been established by insulin assay with oral glucose tolerance and is the basis for this text. (*See Chapter 12.*) Hypoinsulinemia per se with diabetes mellitus glucose tolerance (DMGT) identifies type 1 diabetes, hyperglycemia phase.

Screening for type 1 diabetes.

Screening for type 1 diabetes has been limited. Evidence from type 1 diabetes prevention studies suggest that measurements of islet autoantibodies identify individuals at risk for developing type 1 diabetes. Diabetes Care, January 2010 concluded that widespread clinical testing of asymptomatic low risk individuals cannot be recommended.

Screening for Type 1 diabetes is available.

Hypoinsulin (low insulin) remains the sine qua non of type 1 diabetes.

With the IGT and the NGT, hypoinsulin identifies type 1 diabetes in-situ (occult diabetes), prehyperglycemia. Type 1 diabetes and Type 2 diabetes have their beginning when the blood sugars are normal.

Applying the insulin assay with oral glucose tolerance to ongoing national and international diabetes detection studies especially of the young is a practical application of screening for type 1 and type 2 diabetes. Until the earliest diagnosis of type 2 and type 1 diabetes becomes a diagnostic objective, thereby providing the earliest opportunity for treatment and cure, the worldwide clinical silence of diabetes will continue to be an enigma of international clinical medicine.

Dr. Kenneth H. Brookler in his book review provides a succinct closing for this Preface.

"This wonderful written book is suitable for both the public and for the profession. It is a treasure of knowledge and experience not otherwise available. This work should be required reading for all medical students, endocrinologists, otolaryngologists, and anybody interested in their future – and especially for physicians concerned about their future and that of their patients."

JOSEPH R. KRAFT, M.D.

Preface 2009

DUE TO THE dearth and almost total absence of autopsy experience and/or exposure, physicians and research investigators have been deprived of the opportunity for knowledge of the pathology of type 2 diabetes. MRI and other diagnostic modalities yet to be, are not substitutes for the autopsy, which remains the pillar of medicine.

DIABETES EPIDEMIC and YOU provides extensive autopsy and clinical pathology experience, addressing the pathogenesis of type 2 diabetes. It highlights the history and current application of the oral glucose tolerance with insulin assays in clinical medicine.

The 14,384 oral glucose tolerances with insulin assays are separated according to age, beginning with less than 13 years to 81-90+ years of age. This resource is unequaled in world medical literature.

In recent times, the clinical application of the oral glucose tolerance with insulin assays has been minimal. Many pathologists and most clinicians, including professors from distinguished universities, have little to zero experience with it. In order for their opinions to have creditability regarding the procedure and its interpretation, a randomized personal experience with a thousand procedures would suffice. Once this experience has been achieved, the reproducibility of the oral glucose tolerance with insulin assays will be self-evident.

The pathology of diabetes mellitus occurs in those with normal blood sugars. There are far too many who are told, "Don't worry, your fasting blood sugars are normal." The earliest diagnosis of prediabetes is hyperinsulin, type 2 diabetes identified by insulin assays with normal glucose tolerance. With early diagnosis, the DIABETES EPIDEMIC can be arrested and then reversed.

This is the goal of this book that I share with YOU. Hopefully, it will help you to turn the dream into a reality, i.e. the prevention of the pathology of diabetes mellitus and cardiovascular disease.

Joseph R. Kraft, MD

Diabetes Epidemic and You will alert people worldwide about the importance of the earliest diagnosis and treatment of prediabetes and diabetes. Increased insulins with normal blood sugars in this astonishing experience of 14,384 oral sugar tolerances with insulin assays established the earliest diagnosis. International recognition will, in my opinion, establish Dr. Kraft as the "Father of Insulin Assay" in clinical medicine.

> —Professor Doctor Yotaka Fukuda, MD, PhD
> Department of Otolaryngology and Biophysics
> Escola Paulista de Medicina
> São Paulo, Brasil

Dr. Kraft's quarter century's devoted study of glucose metabolism and blood insulin levels, before its recognition by clinicians, is thoroughly elaborated and clinically correlated in his sentinel monograph. This book presents Dr. Kraft's exceptional cumulative experience with 14,384 oral glucose tolerance tests with insulin assays performed at St. Joseph Hospital, Chicago, between 1972 and 1998, while he was the chairman of the Department of Pathology and Nuclear Medicine. No parallel experience has ever been reported. This volume provides the earliest diagnosis of prediabetes and diabetes—even when the fasting blood sugar levels have been considered to be normal. As the author comments and I agree, "The book should awaken the silent millions with undiagnosed diabetes..."

> —William H. Wehrmacher, MD, FACP, FACC
> Clinical Professor of Medicine and Adjunct Professor of Physiology
> Loyola University of Chicago, Stritch School of Medicine
> Editor: Book review section of the journal, *Comprehensive Therapy*

Contents

Preface 2011		v
Acknowledgements		ix
Introduction		x
Part One	**The Evolution of the Diabetes Epidemic**	**1**
Chapter 1	American Diabetes Association and Department of Health and Human Services Screening Recommendations	3
Chapter 2	Fasting Blood Sugar: What Is Normal?	5
Chapter 3	Diabetes in Ancient Times	8
Chapter 4	Hippocrates: The Father of Medicine	10
Chapter 5	Diabetes History: Sixteenth to Nineteenth Centuries	12
Chapter 6	Discovery of Insulin	15
Chapter 7	The Yalow-Berson Contribution: The Radioimmunoassay of Insulin	17
Chapter 8	The Atomic Energy Act of 1945 And Laboratory Medicine	19
Chapter 9	Oak Ridge Institute of Nuclear Studies	21
Chapter 10	History of the Insulin Assay St. Joseph Hospital, Chicago, Illinois 1972–1998	23
Chapter 11	Normal Fasting Insulin: What Is Normal?	28
Chapter 12	Dynamic Insulin Patterns	31
Chapter 13	The Oral Glucose Tolerance: 1918–2007	45
Chapter 14	Pathology of Type 2 Diabetes	49
Chapter 15	Hyperinsulinemia: Clinical Pathology	54
Chapter 16	Functional Hypoglycemia: Clinical Fact or Fiction?	57

Chapter 17	Gestational Diabetes		60
Chapter 18	C-Reactive Protein		67
Chapter 19	Cholesterol: A Risk Factor for Heart Disease and Diabetes?		69
Chapter 20	Overweight/Obese: A Risk Factor for Heart Disease and Diabetes		71
Chapter 21	Know Your Risk Factors for Heart Disease and Diabetes		74
Chapter 22	The Metabolic Syndrome: What Is It?		77
Chapter 23	Diabetes and Idiopathic Cardiomyopathy		79
Chapter 24	Hyperinsulinemia vs. Insulin Resistance		81
Part Two	**Age Distribution of 14,384 Oral Glucose Tolerances With Insulin Assays**		**83**
Chapter 25	3–13 Age Group		85
Chapter 26	14–20 Age Group		89
Chapter 27	21–30 Age Group		91
Chapter 28	31–40 Age Group		93
Chapter 29	41–50 Age Group		95
Chapter 30	51–60 Age Group		97
Chapter 31	61–70 Age Group		99
Chapter 32	71–80 Age Group		101
Chapter 33	81–90+ Age Group		103
Chapter 34	Diabetes: A Worldwide Plague Facing the Challenge		105

Acknowledgements

WITHOUT KIAN T. Sie, this book would never have materialized. Dr. Sie was the orchestrator of the cumulative data over a 25-year period, which made this book a reality.

My fellow clinical pathologists, Leif Bjornson, Marie Munoz, and Dilip Dharkar, provided me their friendship and support.

Last and not least are the medical technologists during this 25-year period, without whom the 14,384 oral glucose tolerances with insulin assays would not have happened.

A very special thank you to Barbara Loescher at ScriptPerfect, who transferred my writings into perfect script.

Introduction

THE GOAL OF this book is to awaken the silent millions with undiagnosed diabetes to combat the Diabetes Epidemic beginning with you—and I do mean YOU!

In very recent times, the reality of the Diabetes Epidemic has been highlighted by all of the news media. Over 40 million in the U. S. alone and hundreds of millions worldwide already have diabetes and do not know it!

Fasting high blood sugar is diabetes. *Prediabetes* is a term in which the fasting blood sugar is above the "normal" and less than the high fasting sugar of diabetes. Diabetes has a beginning early in life. Genetic studies have not as yet been established and are tools of the future yet to be unveiled. The Center for Disease Control (CDC) reported the following in October of 2006:

- Two million U. S. youths have prediabetes.
- Condition can be reversed.
- Left unchecked may lead to diabetes and heart disease.
- Kids are not the only ones with prediabetes. Many grownups have it, too.

The sugar in your body is carried in your blood. It is essential for life. Without it, you are no more! Your sugar can be accurately measured in your blood. A small sample is taken from you before your breakfast. This measurement is now called your *fasting blood sugar*. Whenever or whatever food you eat, your fasting blood sugar will immediately respond. This is exactly what must happen. All your food is changed by wonderful events within you to become sugar. This now becomes the source of energy and life of every cell of your body. This amazing event does not just happen by itself. It needs a very special hormone that is essential for your cells to utilize the sugar. This hormone is *insulin*.

The terms "blood sugar" and "blood glucose" are one and the same as applied in this book. The oral glucose (sugar) tolerance is simply having the person to be tested—after a fasting blood sugar specimen has been obtained—receive a given amount of sugar in a liquid. Thereafter, at scheduled time intervals, blood specimens for sugar determinations are obtained.

The oral glucose tolerance has been an established procedure for the diagnosis of early diabetes since 1921. The oral glucose tolerance with insulin assays has been a routine procedure at St. Joseph Hospital since 1972. This test has provided the earliest diagnosis of prediabetes and diabetes even when the blood sugars were normal.

The table of contents lists the chapters that highlight the history and current application of the oral glucose tolerance with insulin assays in clinical medicine. The 14,384 oral glucose tolerances with insulin assays are separated according to age. There are nine groups, beginning with 3–13 years of age to the 81–90+ years of age. This constitutes the Part Two section of this book.

This resource of the oral glucose tolerance with insulin assay is unequaled in world medical literature. The earliest diagnosis of prediabetes is hyperinsulin, type 2 diabetes identified by insulin assay with normal glucose tolerance. When coupled with specific therapy, the Diabetes Epidemic will be arrested and then reversed. This is the goal of this book.

If you are concerned about your future, you can find your age group in Part Two. Each group has been further divided into normal glucose tolerance (NGT), impaired glucose tolerance (IGT), and diabetes mellitus glucose tolerance (DMGT). Each of you, upon testing by an oral glucose tolerance, would be in one of these categories.

Following the *Chicago Tribune* report of my presentation, "The Glucose Tolerance Examination: An Obsolete Procedure," read at the Symposium on Radioimmunoassay in Diagnostic Medicine, Annual Convention, American Medical Association, Chicago, Illinois, June 25, 1974, *Newsweek* dispatched a reporter to Chicago to interview me.

The reporter was a skilled young lady with a science background. Her report highlighted the early identification of type 2 diabetes by the oral glucose tolerance with increased insulin. Whenever increased insulins of type 2 diabetes were associated with normal blood sugars, "occult" or "prediabetes" was identified. The report, "New Test for Diabetes," Newsweek, July 29, 1974, page 70, is now historic. It further noted that dietary control in early cases can prevent progression of the disease.

This book, *DIABETES EPIDEMIC and YOU*, is my cumulative experience of 14,384 oral glucose tolerances with insulin assays performed at St. Joseph Hospital, Chicago, Illinois from 1972 to 1998, while I was chairman of the Department of Clinical Pathology and Nuclear Medicine.

Part One

The Evolution of the Diabetes Epidemic

1

AMERICAN DIABETES ASSOCIATION AND DEPARTMENT OF HEALTH AND HUMAN SERVICES SCREENING RECOMMENDATIONS

IN 2002, UNDER the direction of Secretary Tommy Thompson and Francine Kaufman, MD, then President, American Diabetes Association, a panel of the Department of Health and Human Services and the American Diabetes Association (ADA) unveiled recommendations for physicians to begin screening for prediabetes and diabetes by fasting blood glucose or oral glucose tolerance tests, particularly in overweight people 45 and older. Prediabetes, also known as impaired glucose tolerance (IGT) and impaired fasting glucose (IFG), was cited as a serious condition treatable by early diagnosis.

In 2002, the normal fasting blood glucose (FBG) was less than 110 mg/dl. The panel recommended that fasting blood glucose of 110–125 mg/dl be designated impaired and require an oral glucose tolerance test. Fasting blood glucoses ≥126 mg/dl were judged diabetes, provisional. This is an extremely high blood sugar, yet in most instances is free of symptoms. The panel emphasized that most people with prediabetes develop full-blown type 2 diabetes (hyperglycemic phase) within 10 years, with risk of heart disease being increased by 50%. The American Diabetes Association Clinical Practice Recommendations in January 2006 and 2007, *Diabetes Care* Suppl 1, further defined screening for prediabetes and diabetes:

1. Individuals under 45 years of age and overweight, plus if they have any other risk factors for diabetes should be tested.
2. Consistent with the screening recommendations for adults, children and youths at increased risk for the presence or development of type 2 diabetes should be tested.

In 2004 and thereafter to the current time, the "normal" FBG has been designated less than 100 mg/dl. FBGs of 100–125 mg/dl were designated "impaired" and would require an oral glucose tolerance test. FBGs of ≥126 mg/dl were designated "diabetes provisional" and required concurrence on another day.

The ADA Standards for fasting blood glucose mg/dl:

1997–2003	FBG	2004–2007
110	Normal	100
≥110–125	Impaired	≥100–125
≥126	Diabetes (Provisional)	≥126

To what extent physicians have responded to the panel recommendations for screening is not known. What normal fasting blood glucose values the physicians have been utilizing is also unknown. There are two questions you must implicitly ask your doctor:
1. Is my fasting blood sugar normal?
2. If normal, will I ever develop diabetes?

2

FASTING BLOOD SUGAR: WHAT IS NORMAL?

THE QUESTION OF what is normal fasting blood sugar has been asked over and over again. The answer depends upon the experiences of the observers and their time in history:

1925	100 mg/dl (90–120 = normal range)
1968	less than 130 mg/dl
1979	less than 115 mg/dl
1997-2003	less than 110 mg/dl
2004-2007	less than 100 mg/dl

—American Diabetes Association Clinical Practice Recommendations, *Diabetes Care* Suppl 1: January 2003–2007.

Blood sugar measurements in 1925 were performed on a Folin-Wu filtrate. This was the state of the art of clinical laboratory medicine for many years. This technique contained trace amounts of other substances. For historical interest, I refer you to the following classic text: *Clinical Diagnosis by Laboratory Methods: A Working Manual of Clinical Pathology* by James Campbell Todd, MD, Professor of Clinical Pathology, School of Medicine, University of Colorado, 5th ed. (W. B. Saunders Company, 1925) p. 369.

From 1950 on, more precise and specific analytic methods for glucose determinations have been employed. The term "blood" glucose and "plasma" glucose specimens in this presentation are synonymous. The glucose determinations for the 14,384 oral glucose tolerances were from the blood plasma.

Table 1. Fasting Blood Glucose less than 110 milligrams per deciliter in 14,384 Oral Glucose Tolerance Tests Designated Normal (NGT), Impaired (IGT), and Diabetes Mellitus Glucose Tolerance (DMGT).

	NGT (n=9598)	IGT (n=2775)	DMGT (n=2011)
Fasting blood glucose*			
<110 mg/dl	99%	84%	40%
<100 mg/dl	93%	60%	20%
<90 mg/dl	71%	32%	13%
<80 mg/dl	32%	12%	4%
<70 mg/dl	9%	9%	2%
<60 mg/dl	2%	2%	<1%

*To convert glucose values to millimoles per liter, multiply by 0.0551

Dear reader, what is your fasting blood sugar? Please see Table 1. The 14,384 oral glucose tolerances are designated normal glucose tolerance (NGT), impaired glucose tolerance (IGT), and diabetes mellitus glucose tolerance (DMGT). The fasting blood glucoses of less than 110 mg/dl to less than 60 mg/dl have been correlated with each category. You may take poetic license and place yourself into one of the three oral glucose tolerance categories based on your fasting blood sugar. You will fit into one of them.

In the absence of high risk for diabetes and in accordance with ADA criteria (2007), those with normal fasting blood glucose, i.e., less than 100 mg/dl, would not be considered prediabetes or diabetes candidates. They would, therefore, not be subject to an oral glucose tolerance 75–g load and would thereby remain undiagnosed and potentially untreated.

The oral glucose tolerance (100–g glucose load) with insulin assays were performed at St. Joseph Hospital, Chicago, Illinois. The procedure was part of the Department's research and development program, and became a routine procedure in 1972. The persons tested were patients of the medical staff. They were submitted to identify or rule out prediabetes or diabetes. In Table 1, 40 percent of the diabetes mellitus glucose tolerances (DMGT) had fasting blood sugars less than 110 mg/dl, and 20 percent or 402 persons of the

2,011 had fasting blood sugars less than 100 mg/dl. If your fasting blood sugar is less than 100 mg/dl ("normal" 2006–2007), you could possibly still be like one of the 402 diabetics and *not know it*.

The *New England Journal of Medicine*, October 6, 2005, featured a very timely article entitled "Normal Fasting Blood Glucose Levels" by A. Tiroch et al. in the Israeli Diabetes Research Group, *N Engl J Med* 353:1459–62. The background for their research was the question of whether fasting blood glucose levels within the recently defined range of less than 100 mg/dl could independently predict type 2 diabetes in young adults. Their data was obtained from blood measurements, physical examinations, and medical and lifestyle information from men in the Israel Defense Force who were 26–45 years of age. A total of 208 incident cases of type 2 diabetes occurred during the follow up (1992–2004) among the 13,163 subjects who had baseline fasting blood glucose levels of less than 100 mg/dl. The study concluded that higher fasting glucose levels within the normoglycemic range, i.e., less that 100 mg/dl, constitute an independent risk factor for type 2 diabetes among young men, and that the sustaining of normal fasting blood glucose levels did not exclude the subsequent occurrence of type 2 diabetes.

A question you may now ask is what is diabetes? The subsequent chapters will answer that question.

3

Diabetes in Ancient Times

TO GAIN AN appreciation of increased insulin (hyperinsulinemia) and increased glucose of diabetes mellitus, one must begin with an awareness of the history of diabetes. In the Ebers papyrus dating back to the seventeenth dynasty (1650–5132 BC), there is testimony to a long history of diabetes before it was ever given a name. This papyrus was found in a tomb in Thebes in 1862 and named after the Egyptologist George Ebers. It contained descriptions of various diseases, including a polyuric state (frequent urination) resembling diabetes mellitus, as we now know it. The papyrus also contained a four–day treatment course consisting of a decoction of bones, wheat, grain, grit, green lead, and earth. This has been described as being no more bizarre and no less successful than that which had been prescribed over the next thousand years.

We must never forget, however, that whenever the cause and effect of a clinical condition is not definitive, speculative creativity results under the guise of research. This is true in the present as well as in ancient times.

The term "diabetes," which is Ionian Greek and means "to run through" or a "siphon," was first used by Aretaeus of Cappadocia in the second century AD as a generic description for a condition causing increased urine output. Aretaeus described this condition accurately, which is immediately recognizable today. His description is so remarkable that I will now cite it in part from Papaspros, N. S. ed. 1964. *The History of Diabetes Mellitus*, 2nd ed. Stuttgart: Georg Thieme Verlag.

> Diabetes is a dreadful affliction, not very frequent among men, being a melt down of the flesh and limbs into urine. The patient never stops making water and the flow is incessant, like opening an aqueduct. Life is short, unpleasant and painful, thirst unquenchable, drinking excessive and disproportionate to the large quantity of urine, for yet more urine is passed.

One cannot stop them either from drinking or making water. If for a while they abstain from drinking, their mouths become parched and their bodies dry; the viscera seem scorched up; the patients are affected by nausea, restlessness, and a burning thirst, and within a short time, they expire.

The Roman physician, Claudius Galenus (Galen: 125–199 AD), like Aretaeus, thought diabetes to be a rare disease and apparently had encountered only two cases. Galen employed alternative terms for diabetes, including "diarrhea urinosa" and "dipsatos," the latter emphasizing the cardinal symptoms of excessive thirst and drinking. The association of *polyuria* with a sweet-tasting substance in the urine was first reported in the Sanskrit literature dating from the fifth to sixth centuries AD. The urine of the polyuric patients was described as tasting like honey, being sticky to the touch and strongly attracting ants and flies.

It is most interesting that the Indian physicians of this time suggested two forms of diabetes—one affecting older, fatter people and the other thin people who did not survive long. During this era, Chinese and Japanese physicians also described this polyuric condition with the sweetness of urine which attracted small animals, including dogs. They also observed that these individuals were prone to develop boils, a condition which even today prevails in those with diabetes.

The fact that diabetic urine tasted sweet was subsequently emphasized in Arabic medical texts during the centuries when Arabic medicine was at its peak of achievement. The most influential Arabic contributor to medicine was Avicenna (980–1037 AD), whose standing in both Islam and Christendom was equal to that of Galen. Until the mid-seventeenth century, the curriculum of the Christian universities, including those in the British Isles, was based on Avicenna's writings. He described accurately the clinical features of diabetes. He specifically mentioned two complications of the disease—gangrene and the collapse of sexual function—both of which prevail today worldwide in the diagnosed and undiagnosed diabetic population. Both conditions must have been of significant incidence to have been judged worthy of note by Avicenna. While the gangrene was objective, the sexual dysfunction was totally subjective. Sexual dysfunction, now known as *penile erectile dysfunction* (PED), must have been of grave concern to the men at the time of Avicenna, just as it is today to men worldwide.

PED is a personal physical manifestation of hyperinsulinemia, type 2 diabetes, even in those with "normal" fasting blood sugars. All PED must be considered hyperinsulinemia, type 2 diabetes until proven otherwise by oral glucose tolerance with insulin assays.

4

Hippocrates: The Father of Medicine

THE PURPOSE OF the Egyptian papyri was to provide physicians with instruction of methods to be applied in curing diseases and in preparing medicine, with no particular emphasis or discussion of differential diagnosis or etiology. It remained for the ancient Greeks to initiate this gigantic step and to endeavor to establish a theoretical basis for treatment. The first instance of medicine deserving of the adjective "scientific" was in ancient Greece. It was connected with the name Hippocrates.

The Alexandrian accounts of the life of Hippocrates are rich in detail, noting that he was born in the year 460 BC, descended from Hercules as well as from Asclepious. Hippocrates studied medicine and philosophy with famous teachers, and traveled over the entire Greek world. He died at an advanced age, estimated to be at or near 100 years. His tomb could still be seen in the second century AD, according to Celcus Cornelius (circa AD 30). A medical writer of renown, Hippocrates was as eminent for his eloquence as for his knowledge.

There is one saying that has achieved universal use, and only a few who quote it today are aware that Hippocrates was referring to the art of the physician. It has been referenced as the first of his aphorisms.

"Life is short and
the art is long;
the occasion fleeting;
experience fallacious and
judgment difficult."

The Hippocrates figure as the legendary Father of Medicine soon replaced the historical Hippocrates. More than sixty books or manuscripts are assumed to have originated from Hippocrates' time, i.e., fourth and fifth centuries, BC. Presumably they were compiled in the second century AD as *Corpus Hippocraticum*. This now goes by the name *Hippocratic Collection*.

It remains even to this day an important compendium of the medical science of antiquity. Specific symptoms of diabetes are not identified.

The writings of Hippocrates are truly exceptional on physician behavior. The Hippocratic Oath is the known document associated most widely with his name. This famous testament contained both affirmations and prohibitions targeted for the physicians of his time, when abortion and assisted suicide prevailed:

> "I will neither give a deadly drug to anybody if asked for it.
> Similarly, I will not give a woman an abortion remedy.
> In purity and holiness, I will guard my life and my art."

The earliest reference to the oath occurs in the first century AD. Later, it was adapted to Christianity by substituting God, Christ, and/or saints for the name Asclepious and his family. Gradually, medical students for centuries have stood to swear to the provisions of this oath. Self-evident today in the practice of medicine is the present and ongoing, never-ending, worldwide need of a continuous renewal of moral and virtuous principles based upon natural law unaltered by secularism.

The emphasis that Hippocrates placed on nutrition must not be overlooked. In the oath, he further states, "I will apply dietetic measures for the benefit of the sick according to my ability and judgment." Based on his recognition of the importance of nutrition as a method of treatment in medicine, Hippocrates has also been credited as the Father of Dietetics.

For many succeeding generations, Hippocrates was the ideal physician. Several hundred years later, Galen, a distinguished Roman physician, venerated Hippocrates as one "... who with purity and holiness lived his life and practiced his art." I have previously referred to Galen as the one who employed the alternative terms of diarrhea urinosa and dipsakos for diabetes. Galen is a most interesting person. At the beginning of his career, he had been a physician to gladiators. Later, he became the personal physician to the emperor, Marcus Aurelius. Galen acknowledged that Hippocrates was truly a man of virtue.

5

DIABETES HISTORY: SIXTEENTH TO NINETEENTH CENTURIES

SEVERAL CENTURIES APPARENTLY elapsed before European physicians made observations that diabetic urine was sugary. The sixteenth-century Swiss physician, von Hohenheim (1493–1591), who humbly accorded himself the name "Paracelsus" in self-recognition of his own scientific achievements, reported that diabetic urine contained an abnormal substance which remained as a white powder after evaporation. He concluded that this substance was a salt and that, in diabetes, this was due to a deposition of salt in the kidneys causing "thirst" of the kidneys and hence polyuria.

It was not until the seventeenth century that Thomas Willis (1621–1675) made reference to the sweet taste of the diabetic urine and thereby duplicated the observations which had appeared over a thousand years before in the Egyptian and Eastern writings. Dr. Willis made several other astute observations about diabetes. He wrote that diabetes had been rare in classical times, "... but now, we meet with examples ... I may say daily of this disease ... wherefore the urine of the sick is so wonderfully sweet ... or hath an honied taste...." Willis continued: "As to what belongs the cure ... it seems a hard thing in this disease to draw propositions for curing, for that its causes lies so deeply hid, and hath its origin so deep and remote." Hundreds of years later, into this twenty-first century, the cure has not yet been fully unveiled.

Another celebrated physician of the seventeenth century was Dr. Thomas Sydenham (1624–1684) who speculated that diabetes was a systemic disease in which the blood contained products of incomplete digestion of food, and its non-absorbed residue had to be excreted. About a century later, Dr. Matthew Dobson (1735–1784), a Liverpool physician, published in 1776 a series of experiments on his nine patients with diabetes that the blood serum as well as their urine contained a substance with a sweet taste. Furthermore, he proved that the substance was sugar. He concluded that this had previously existed in the serum rather than being formed in the kidney. This was the first evidence that diabetes might be a generalized disorder.

A few years after Dr. Dobson's important paper, another English physician, Dr. John Rollo, published his study on two cases of diabetes (1809) in which he was the first to use the adjective "mellitus." This word was derived from the Latin and Greek roots for "honey." It was used to distinguish the condition of diabetes with its characteristic sweet urine from another polyuric disease in which sugar was absent in the urine. The Latin term *insipidus* was applied to this condition and designated "diabetes insipidus." This disease, which still prevails today, has no relationship to diabetes mellitus. Dr. Rollo made another significant observation. He reported the greater association of cataracts in some diabetics and the notation of the odor of acetone (which he compared to like decaying apples) on the breath of some diabetic persons. The latter is now known as "ketosis."

In 1855, French physiologist Claude Bernard demonstrated that the sugar that appears in the urine of diabetics was stored in the liver in the form of glycogen. Coma was first recognized as a complication of diabetes by Dr. W. Prout (1785–1859), an English physician at Guy's Hospital. An American ophthalmologist, Dr. H. D. Noyes, in 1869 published a report that a form of retinitis occurred in glycosuric patients.

In 1869, while working on his doctorate dissertation, Paul Langerhans (1847–1888) had noted small clusters of cells in his tissue preparations of pancreas which were separable from the surrounding exocrine and ductal tissue. Langerhans simply described these structures without speculating in his thesis as to their possible function.

In 1874, Professor A. Kussmal (1821–1902) of Freiberg University in Germany described the "air hunger" of ketoacidosis in diabetes. Even to this day, very rapid breathing implies a condition known as metabolic acidosis occurring in diabetes and is named Kussmal Breathing. He had observed, by gentle palpation, increased pressure within the jugular veins occurred upon deep inspiration and returned to normal upon exhaling. Failure to return to normal he judged to be indicative of increased venous pressure throughout the body. Dr. Kussmal reported that the increased venous pressure could be identified before the clinical symptoms—mainly edematous swelling of the legs, increased fluid (ascites) in the abdominal cavity, and congestion of the liver—were identified. This observation has been named the Kussmal Sign.

In 1890, Oskar Minkowski and Josef von Mering reported their experimental work, which firmly established the role of the pancreas in causing diabetes. The experiment was performed at the University of Strasbourg. The pancreas of a dog was removed to determine whether it was essential for life. After the operation, the animal unexpectedly displayed the typical signs of severe diabetes. The dog was hyperglycemic and glycosuric. The dog was now diabetic. The long-sought answer regarding the structural origin of diabetes was now answered.

In 1893, Edouard Laguesse (1861–1927) suggested that the clumps of cells described by Langerhans be named the Islets of Langerhans, and that they might constitute the endocrine tissue of the pancreas. This concept was continued by a Belgian physician, Dr. Jean de Meyer, who in 1909 gave the name "insulin" (Latin *insula* or island) to the glucose-lowering hormone. At that time, the existence of a glucose-lowering hormone was still hypothetical. Dr. de Meyer had postulated that this hormone was produced by the islet tissue. Insulin, therefore, became a substance, an entity, which was named before it was actually discovered.

Minkowski and Von Mering's discovery in 1890 that dogs developed severe diabetes immediately after pancreatectomy stimulated the idea of treating diabetes with pancreatic tissue. Many researchers reported negative or inconclusive results. Some claimed to have isolated pancreatic extracts which could reduce the sugar in the urine and the glucose in the blood when given to diabetic patients. However none could repeat their experimental work nor convince the medical community of their results.

6

Discovery of Insulin

THE DISCOVERY OF insulin with clinical application is a story in itself. The following is a very brief review of the highlights leading to one of the most dramatic impacts in the entire ongoing history of medicine.

In 1920, Dr. Frederick Grant Banting (1891–1941), a practicing physician and surgeon in London, Ontario, was convinced that if one could ligate the ducts of the pancreas, it would cause the gland to shrink and degenerate, leaving the Islets of Langerhans. An extract of the remaining tissue, hopefully containing the islets, would be injected into a diabetic person. If the sugar spilling into the urine would be immediately relived, Dr. Banting postulated that this would prove his hypothesis that insulin came from the islets. Dr. Banting convinced J. W. Macleod, PhD (1876–1935), of the merit of his concept. In 1921, Dr. Macleod provided Banting with the experimental facilities plus a medical student as an assistant, Charles H. Best (1899–1978). Their initial experiments were only partially successful. Finally, after much discouragement, Dr. Banting requested help. Dr. Macleod invited a skilled biochemist, James B. Collip, PhD (1892–1962) to join the team. Even though their experimental results were not conclusive, Banting and Best presented their preliminary report at a meeting of the American Physiological Society on December 30, 1921. The paper was severely criticized.

Meanwhile, Dr. Collip, working independently, developed an extraction technique which removed the toxic contaminates of the crude extract of Banting and Best. Nevertheless, Banting and Best, convinced of the quality of their extract, gave it to a fourteen-year-old boy dying of diabetes in Toronto General Hospital on January 12, 1922. It failed! On January 23, 1922, a separate extract made by Dr. Collip was given to the same fourteen-year-old boy. The results were immediate and dramatic. Collip's extract reduced the blood sugar to normal, abolished the excretion of sugar in the urine, and ended the ketonuria. Hereby, the use of insulin in the treatment of diabetes mellitus was inaugurated. That fourteen-year-old patient had *juvenile dia-*

betes, i.e., he was severely deficient in producing his own insulin in sufficient amounts. This form of diabetes is now designated type 1 diabetes mellitus. The Collip technique was crude, inconsistent, and capable of only limited production. These problems were not solved until there was collaboration with the chemists of the Eli Lilly Company of Indiana. A commercially viable extraction technique involving isoelectric precipitation was developed. By October 1923, insulin became widely available in North America and Europe.

In 1923, the Nobel Committee, with unprecedented promptness, awarded Banting and Macleod the prize in physiology/medicine for the discovery of insulin. The controversy over who should also have been recognized was never officially resolved. However, the formal winners shared their prize money with Best and Collip.

Thus we come to the end of an era and the beginning of another.

History references and suggested readings:
1. Hutchins, R. M., ed. 1952. *Great Books of the Western World*, vol. 10. Chicago: Encyclopedia Britannica.
    a) Hippocrates and Galen, p. 131
    b) Aphorisms, *xi*
2. Lyons, A. S., and R. J. Petrocelli, eds. 1987. *Medicine: An Illustrated History*. New York: Abrams.
    a) Ancient Egypt, pp. 77–104
    b) Medicine in Hippocratic times, pp. 195–215
    c) Medical sects and The Center at Alexandria, pp. 219–230
    d) Galen, pp. 250–261
    e) Ancient India, pp. 105–120
3. Pickup, J. C., and G. Williams, eds. 1997. "History of Diabetes Mellitus." In *Textbook of Diabetes*, 2nd ed., vol. 1. (London: Blackwell Science), 1–21.

7

THE YALOW-BERSON CONTRIBUTION: THE RADIOIMMUNOASSAY OF INSULIN

INSULIN WAS PREPARED from the pancreas glands of cows and pigs. It became of clinical concern that, over a period of time, there was an unexplained increased requirement of the insulin units needed per day by the patients. This increased requirement was arbitrarily defined as "insulin resistance." It was applied whenever a daily requirement of 200 units or more was necessary to maintain normal metabolic stability. Fortunately, the incidence of insulin resistance requiring very high doses of insulin greater than 1,000–25,000 units per day are now rare.

A quantitative measurement of the patient's insulin was not yet available but was being sought by many. It must be noted that the clinical concept at that time was that diabetes mellitus was total or eventually a total insulin deficiency. There are some who hold to this concept even today, which I will subsequently address.

In the 1950s, Solomon A. Berson, MD, Director of Radioisotope Unit, Veterans Administration Hospital, Bronx, NY, and Rosalyn Yalow, PhD, a physicist also at the V. A. hospital, pioneered the study of the behavior of iodine-131 labeled insulin. In 1951, J. Bornstein and R. D. Lawrence published a bioassay technique demonstrating insulin in a small number of diabetic patients (*Br Med J* 2:144–5). Their bioassay and other similar insulin bioassay procedures were neither practical nor applicable to clinical medicine. As a consequence, they received little attention. Yalow and Berson's study of radioactive labeled insulin (iodine-131 labeled insulin) made several important observations that led to the development of a radioimmunoassay for plasma insulin. (Yalow, R. S., and S. A. Berson. 1960. Immunoassay of endogenous plasma insulin in man. *J Clin Invest* 30:1157–75.) (Yalow, R. S., and S. A Berson. 1960. Plasma insulin concentrations in nondiabetic and early diabetic subjects. *Diabetes* 9:254–60.) They observed that when patients were treated with insulin, insulin-binding antibodies were formed to the injected insulin. This accounted for the so-called "insulin resistance." It was this principle of antigen-antibody reaction that Yalow and Berson applied to their iodine-131 labeled insulin studies. They produced insulin antibodies by injecting guinea pigs with insulin. They subsequently observed that unlabeled-insulin displaced radioactive-labeled insulin from the insulin antibody. This became the basis of radioimmunoassay.

For this procedure development in analytic clinical chemistry, Dr. Yalow shared with others a 1977 Nobel Prize. Dr. Yalow also shared her financial prize with Dr. Berson, who was her husband.

8

The Atomic Energy Act of 1945 and Laboratory Medicine

THE ATOMIC ENERGY Act of 1945 decreed that atomic energy was to be applied and utilized in medicine. A requirement of the Act stated that before a physician could be allowed utilization of any radioactive material, he must first be certified by a PhD physicist, primarily for safety training regarding exposure to radioactivity. The intent of the Atomic Energy Act was handcuffed by this requirement. First of all, the amount of radiation exposure with radioisotopes was minute. Secondly, the physicists were of limited number and were the first to acknowledge their lack of knowledge in matters of medicine. Modification of this requirement occurred by authority of the Atomic Energy Commission (AEC) formed in 1947.

In 1955, the College of American Pathologists conjointly with the American Society of Clinical Pathologists initiated a workshop on atomic energy safety, in cooperation with the Atomic Energy Commission. I was privileged to attend this workshop, which was small in the number of participants. It was under the direction of Oscar B. Hunter, Jr., MD, director of the Oscar B. Hunter Memorial Laboratory and Professor of Clinical Pathology at Georgetown University in Washington, DC. Upon completion of the workshop, the AEC licensed each of the participants to obtain radioisotope material available at that time for clinical laboratory testing. The utilization of radioisotopes was an exciting new dimension in laboratory medicine. It was an adjunct to the clinical chemistry already in place. As an extended tool of analytical chemistry, the utilization of radioisotopes yielded unprecedented accuracy, specificity, and reproducibility in clinical laboratory medicine.

Without question, the leading clinical pathologist into this new frontier of diagnostic laboratory medicine was Dr. Oscar B. Hunter. At that time, I was Pathologist and Director of Laboratories at St. Francis Hospital in

Peoria, Illinois, where we had been provided a scintillation gamma counter for radioisotope testing. I say *we*, because Ernie P. Elzi, MD—my co-director and very best friend—and I began our adventure into radioassay medicine together.

9

Oak Ridge Institute of Nuclear Studies

IN 1957, MARSHAL Brucer, MD, Medical Director of the Oak Ridge Institute of Nuclear Studies (ORINS) in Oak Ridge, Tennessee, initiated a comprehensive program in radioisotope technology. The faculty was from the Institute, all of whom were experts and pioneers in their fields. The course was two weeks, with a separation of three months between the first and second week. It was a five-day program, 7:00 a.m. to 9:00 p.m., with lectures and hands-on workshops. The purpose of the three-month separation was to give each of us an opportunity to apply what we had learned and hopefully to share our experiences in the next session. The number of participants in this program was limited to 20, and I was fortunate to have been included. Like me, all participants were clinical pathologists who had previously obtained the basic AEC licensure. Dr. Brucer, who was a physician with a specialty in medical radiation physics, directed his programs to clinical pathologists for very definite reasons:

1. Radiologists were not basically trained in standardizations and quality control in laboratory medicine.
2. Clinical pathologists, by their very essence, were so trained, and it remains the core of the specialty even today.
3. Radioisotope procedures are laboratory examinations.

The labeling of red blood cells for identification of sub-clinical hemolytic anemias, the labeling of vitamin B-12 for the identification of pernicious anemia, and oleic acid labeling for malabsorption studies were all laboratory procedures. These were the first of the many radioassay procedures that followed. The one test that was not a laboratory procedure was the external counting of radioactivity from radioactive-labeled iodine emitted from the thyroid gland for the determination of hyperthyroidism. Whereas iodine is an essential metabolite of the thyroid gland, it was quite logical, therefore, that radioactive-labeled iodine would be captured by the thyroid gland. The emission of radioactivity within the thyroid gland could thereby be measured over the thyroid gland area. Theoretically, therefore, the external counting by an appropriate gamma-ray scintillation counter could identify normal and/or the increased uptake of hyperthyroidism.

This procedure was initially performed within departments of radiology. It is important to know that the gamma-ray emission of radioisotopes has a different spectrum than that of the x-ray emission. The iodine uptake via radioassay is not an x-ray emission examination. What frustrated Dr. Brucer without end was the total failure of departments of radiology, irrespective of their locations, to employ standardized procedures. In the absence thereof, the results in one institution were devoid of relative value in other institutions. Without standardization and quality control, these procedures in the departments of radiology, according to Dr. Brucer, were virtually worthless.

A highlight of the ORINS program was that it gave a preview of organ imaging by external counting of radioisotopes. They demonstrated that images could be produced on Polaroid film, photographic paper, and x-ray film by the external counting of radioactivity. They further demonstrated that by utilizing an iodine crystal varying from one to four inches in diameter, a highly sensitive detection unit was available. The iodine crystal has its peak sensitivity at 140 keV. This means that any radioisotope whose peak activity is at or near the 140 keV becomes an ideal match with the crystal detector, thereby achieving optimal efficiency. Radioactive iodine-131 with a keV of 145 fulfills this criterion perfectly.

The first radioisotope organ imaging was the thyroid gland. Under standardized conditions, the crystal was to be moved at a controlled rate over the thyroid gland area. The term "scan" was now being introduced into medical usage. We must now move on to St. Joseph Hospital in Chicago, Illinois.

10

History of the Insulin Assay
St. Joseph Hospital, Chicago, Illinois
1972–1998

FROM 1965 TO 1978, I was a member of the clinical faculty of the Department of Pathology at the University of Illinois, School of Medicine, Chicago Campus. This was during the tenure of Professor Cecil Krakower, MD, the chairman of the Department of Pathology. One afternoon a week during the school year, I would be assigned 25–30 second-year students to discuss and review their microscopic pathology slides. Dr. Krakower's emphasis on basic pathology was reflected year after year in the National Board Examinations where his students were always in the top percentile. In 1967, Dr. Krakower assigned me the lecture subject "Diabetes," to be given the following year to the sophomore class of 200+ students. This was an interesting challenge, which I readily accepted.

In my review of the world literature on diabetes, I encountered the now-famous work of R. S. Yalow and S. A. Berson, Immunoassay of Endogenous Plasma Insulin in Man. 1960. *J Clin Invest* 30:1157. It was not until 1970 that Pharmacia Diagnostics AB, in Uppsala, Sweden, made available their product, Pharmacia Insulin RIA, based upon World Health Organization standards for the quantitative measurement of insulin in serum. When this product became available to us with regularity, the insulin assay was applied to our oral glucose tolerance examinations. It became our routine procedure in 1972. The insulin assay became a part of the Department's research and development program.

In 1972, the adventure of the insulin assay with the oral glucose tolerance (100-g load) began. The following are presentations and publications that highlighted this adventure:

1972
- ⇒ 500 Tolerances.
- ⇒ Confirmed Yalow and Berson's findings of increased insulin (hyperinsulin) in their 111 persons, diabetic and nondiabetic, tested by the 100-g 3-h oral glucose tolerance with their radioimmunoassay for insulin. Their insulin responses were unclassified.
- ⇒ Identified and classified five distinct dynamic insulin patterns: normal pattern (euinsulin) associated with normal glucose tolerance; three patterns of increased insulin (hyperinsulin) associated with type 2 diabetes; and a low response pattern (hypoinsulin) associated with
- ⇒ type 1 diabetes, potential.

1973
- ⇒ 1000 Tolerances
- ⇒ "Glucose Tolerance with Insulin Assay." Read at Chicago Pathology Society Spring Meeting, 1973. Published in *Chicago Medicine.*

1974
- ⇒ 2,557 Tolerances
- ⇒ "Glucose Insulin Tolerance: A Routine Laboratory Tool Enhancing Diabetes Detection." *Radioassay: Clinical Concepts,* Symposium on Radioimmunoassay held in Washington, DC, January 28–29, 1974. (Published by G. D. Searle & Co., Skokie, Illinois), 91–106.

1974
- ⇒ 3,000 Tolerances
- ⇒ "The Glucose Tolerance Examination: An Obsolete Procedure." Read at Symposium on Radioimmunoassay in Diagnostic Medicine Annual Convention, American Medical Association. Chicago, Illinois, June 25, 1974.

1974
- ⇒ *Chicago Tribune.* Science Editor. "Report on glucose/insulin tolerance presentation." American Medical Association meeting, Chicago, Illinois, June 26, 1974.

1974
- ⇒ *Newsweek.* Medicine Section. "New Test for Diabetes." July 29, 1974, p. 70.

1975
⇒ Detection of diabetes mellitus in-situ (occult diabetes). February 1975. *Lab Med* 6(2):10–22. (3,650 tolerances)

1975
⇒ "Diabetes Mellitus Phase Identification. A New Dimension of Emphasis in the Early Diagnostic/Therapeutic Management with Therapeutic Intervention Potential." Read at Symposium on Radioimmunoassay in Diagnostic Medicine Annual Convention, American Medical Association. Atlantic City, New Jersey, June 15, 1975.

1975
⇒ Kraft, J. R. and R. A. Nosal. 1975. Insulin values and diagnosis of diabetes. *Lancet* 1:637. (Letter to the Editor.)

1979
⇒ Kraft, J. R. "Glucose/Insulin Tolerance Testing for the Prospective Management of Diabetes/Atherosclerosis with Prime Focus on Childhood." In U. P. Merten and J. Linder, eds. *Pathology: A Medical Specialty*. Proceedings of the Tenth Trienniel World Congress of Anatomic and Clinical Pathology. Rio de Janeiro, September 25–29, 1978. World Association of Societies of Pathology 1979, Cologne, West Germany, pp. 608–11.

1983
⇒ Kraft, J. R. 1983. "Insulin and Glucagon." In B. Rothfeld, ed. *Nuclear Medicine in Vitro*. 2nd ed. (Philadelphia: J. B. Lippincott), 211–223.

1988
⇒ Kraft, J. R. 1988. "Insulin assay diabetic state identification, a specific diagnostic tool of the noninsulin dependent diabetic state, a metabolic disorder." In C. F. Claussen, M. V. Kirtane, and K. Schlitter, eds. *Vertigo, Nausea, Tinnitus, and Hypoacusia in Metabolic Disorders*. Amsterdam: Elsevier), 503-06.

1990
⇒ Kraft, J. R. "Hyperinsulinemia/insulin Resistance: The New Gold Standard of Gestational Diabetes Diagnosis; Gestational Diabetes, a

Distinct Clinical Entity." Rudolph Holmes Memorial Lecture, Chicago Gynecological Society, February 16, 1990, Chicago, Illinois.

1990

⇒ Kraft, J. R. April/June 1990. Insulin Assay Diabetic State Identification. A review of 14,000+ glucose/insulin tolerance examinations. *The Proceedings of the Institute of Medicine of Chicago* 43(2):34.

1990

⇒ Kraft, J. R. and K. T. Sie. 1990. Hyperinsulin/insulin resistant NIDDM state identification; a practical screening procedure. *Diabetes* 39 Suppl: 69S.

1992

⇒ Kraft, J. R. 1992. Hyperinsulinemia (Insulin Resistance), the Diagnostic Identifier of Gestational Diabetes Mellitus. Symposium on Gestational Diabetes, Professor Doctor P. A. M. Weise, Director, University of Graz, Austria.

1992

⇒ Kraft, J. R. "Hyperinsulinemia, a defined marker of in-situ NIDDM and associated metabolic disorders. A review of 15,000+ glucose/insulin tolerance examinations." In C. F. Clausen, M. V. Kirtane, and D. Schneider, eds. *Proceedings of the NES*, Volume XX. Bad Kissingen, Germany, 27–29 March 1992, (Hamburg: Werner Rudat & Co., 1994), 569–76.

1995

⇒ Kraft, J. R. "An Early Metabolic Marker of Idiopathic Tinnitus and Other Neurootological Disorders." Presented July 14, 1995, Fifth International Tinnitus Seminar, July 12–15, 1995, Portland, Oregon, USA.

1995

⇒ Kraft, J. R. and K. T. Sie. "Fasting Hyperinsulinemia: Diagnostic Parameters Applicable to Neurootological Equilibriometric and Related Metabolic Disorders." In C. F. Clausen, M. V. Kirtane, and D. Schneider, eds. *Proceedings of the NES*, Volume XXI. Presented June 2–6, 1993 in Linköping, Sweden (Hamburg: Werner Rudat & Co., 1995), 303–07.

1995

⇒ Kraft, J. R. and K. T. Sie. 1995. "Functional Hypoglycemia: Clinical fact or fiction clarification by glucose/insulin tolerance, hyperinsulinemia identification." In C. F. Clausen, M. V. Kirtane, and D. Schneider, eds. *Proceedings of the NES*, XXI:309–11.

1997

⇒ Kraft, J. R. 1997. "IMx (Abbott) Immunoassay of Insulin: A Practical Alternative to RIA Hyperinsulinemia Identification in Idiopathic Neurootology and Other Hyperinsulin Metabolic Disorders." Presented at the Twenty-fourth Ordinary Congress of the Neurootological and Equilibriometric Society, Haifa, Israel, April 6–10, 1997. *Int Tinnitus J* 3(2):113–16.

1998

⇒ Kraft, J. R. 1998. Hyperinsulinemia: Merging history with idiopathic tinnitus, vertigo and hearing loss. *Int Tinnitus J* 4(2):127-30.

2008

⇒ Kraft, J.R. *Diabetes Epidemic and You, Should Everyone Be Tested?*, Victoria, B.C., Canada, Trafford Publishing 2008

2009

⇒ Kraft, J.R., Wehrmacher W.H. *Diabetes – A Silent Disorder*, Comp. Ther. 2009: 35:155-159

2011

⇒ Kraft, J.R., Wehrmacher W.H. *Earliest Diagnosis of Diabetes* – Not available by fasting blood sugar nor by glycated hemoglobin. Comp Ther. 2011, Publication Pending

11

Normal Fasting Insulin: What Is Normal?

THE RADIOIMMUNOASSAY OF insulin opened an unexplored avenue into clinical laboratory medicine as related to diabetes mellitus. In the 1970s, there was early evaluation of fasting insulins in diabetic persons. Just as the fasting blood glucose for decades had been the cornerstone in the diagnosis and management of diabetes, it was hoped that fasting insulins would be of equal or even of greater importance. However, clinical investigations soon identified that fasting insulin levels were indistinguishable in diabetic and nondiabetic persons.

Please see Table 2. The material in Table 2 is unprecedented and unequaled in the world of medical literature. The 14,384 subjects were healthy persons submitted by their physicians for oral glucose tolerance with insulin assays, 100-g glucose load. This was for the purpose of excluding or identifying diabetes mellitus. The age span was from the very young (less than 14 years of age) to the elderly (greater than 80 years of age). In Table 2, the fasting insulins in the diabetes mellitus glucose tolerances (DMGT) are indistinguishable from those with impaired glucose tolerance (IGT) and those with normal glucose tolerance (NGT). The fasting insulins do not differentiate one type of tolerance response from another.

Table 2. Fasting Insulin Distribution in 14,384 Oral Glucose Tolerances with Insulin Assays Designated Normal (NGT), Impaired (IGT), and Diabetes Mellitus Glucose Tolerance (DMGT).

Microunits*	NGT (N=9598)	IGT (N=2775)	DMGT (N=2011)
0-10	53%	43%	33%
11-15	23%	19%	19%
16-20	11%	14%	14%
12-30	8%	14%	18%
>30†	5%	10%	16%

* To convert microunits per milliliter to picomoles per liter multiply by 6.
† Fasting insulin greater than 30 microunits per milliliter (>180 picomoles per liter) identified hyperinsulinemia per se.

What is normal fasting insulin? This was the question that faced us in 1972–1973, at the beginning of our study. With our first 1,000 oral glucose tolerances with insulin assays, which included persons of all ages from normal (NGT), impaired (IGT), and diabetes mellitus tolerances (DMGT), the mean fasting insulin was determined. The mean fasting insulin was 14.65 microunits/ml. The standard deviation was plus or minus 5 microunits/ml; thereby, the mean of 14.65 plus or minus 3 standard deviations (i.e., 15 microunits/ml) determined the fasting insulin range of 0–30 microunits/ml. The subsequent 14,384 oral glucose tolerances with insulin assays confirmed the "normal" fasting insulin of 0–30 microunits/ml. In the absence of comparable numbers of oral glucose tolerances with insulin assays, the fasting insulin range remains unprecedented and unequalled.

The question of what is normal fasting insulin has been answered. However, it raises another question which must be addressed. Is there any value in determining the fasting insulin? The answer is yes!! Fasting insulins greater than 30 microunits/ml (the upper boundary of normal) are diagnostic, by themselves, of the marked increase of insulin, which is hyperinsulinemia—type 2 diabetes. However, our cumulative study of 14,384 glucose tolerances with insulin assays have shown that less than 8 percent of those with hyperinsulinemia or type 2 diabetes have fasting insulins greater than 30 microunits/ml. Please see Chapter 12, Dynamic Insulin Patterns.

Reference:
Kraft, J. R. and K. T. Sie. "Fasting Hyperinsulinemia: Diagnostic Parameters Applicable to Neurootological Equilibriometric and Related Metabolic Disorders." In C. F. Clausen, M. V. Kirtane, and D. Schneider, eds. *Proceedings of the NES*, Volume XXI. Presented June 2–6, 1993 in Linköping, Sweden (Hamburg: Werner Rudat & Co., 1995), 303-07.

12

Dynamic Insulin Patterns

JUST AS THE fasting insulin boundaries were initially unknown, the dynamic insulin response to the oral glucose tolerance load was also unknown. Our studies of insulin assay on the first 1,000 oral glucose tolerance examinations (100-g load) included normal glucose tolerances, impaired glucose tolerances, and diabetes mellitus glucose tolerances. The established reporting by graphing the blood-glucose tolerance curves was applied. Corresponding graphing of the insulin response produced dynamic flow patterns.

Insulin patterns of increased insulin (hyperinsulinemia, insulin resistance), normal insulin (euinsulinemia), and low insulin (hypoinsulinemia) were identified. The insulin patterns were unchanged and substantiated in the subsequent publication of 2,500, 3,500, 10,000, and 14,384 oral glucose tolerance with insulin assays. Hyperinsulinemia (insulin resistance) identified type 2 diabetes not only in the diabetes mellitus glucose tolerances but also in the impaired glucose tolerances and the normal glucose tolerances.

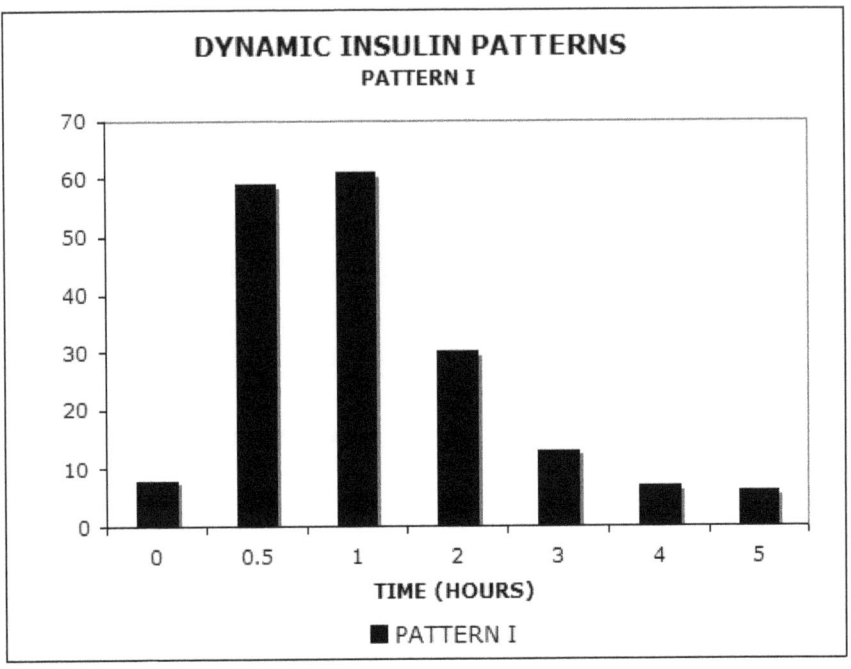

Normal fasting range: 0–30 microunits/ml
½-h or 1-h peak above fasting range
2-h + 3-h sum = less than 60 microunits/ml

N = 2,223

	F	½-h	1-h	2-h	3-h	4-h	5-h
Mean	8	59	61	30	13	7	6

2-h + 3-h sum = 43 microunits/ml

Pattern I is euinsulinemia.

Insulin Pattern I Distribution:
Normal glucose tolerance	2,112 of 9,598	(22%)
Impaired glucose tolerance	83 of 2,775	(3%)
Diabetes mellitus glucose tolerance	28 of 2,011	(1%)

Insulin Pattern I is euinsulinemia. Euinsulinemia identifies nondiabetes with the normal glucose tolerance and with the impaired glucose tolerance.

Twenty-two percent or 2,112 of the 9,598 normal glucose tolerances were euinsulinemia, nondiabetes. *Euinsulinemia with normal glucose tolerance is the true normal glucose tolerance.*

Three percent of the impaired glucose tolerances were euinsulinemia, nondiabetes.

Twenty-eight or 1 percent of the 2,011 diabetes mellitus glucose tolerances were euinsulinemia. Insulin Pattern I is a low insulin response relative to the hyperglycemia of the diabetes mellitus glucose tolerance. The 1 percent with Pattern I and the 8 percent of the diabetes mellitus glucose tolerance with Pattern V (hypoinsulinemia) identify type 1 diabetes potential.

If you have normal insulins with a normal oral glucose tolerance identifying nondiabetes, does it mean that you were never diabetic (hyperinsulinemic) in the past?

No ... it does not!

It demonstrates that you are now doing the right things regarding nutrition, weight control, and exercise. *Keep up the good work*! For your future concerns, please see Chapter 21, "Know Your Risk Factors for Heart Disease and Diabetes."

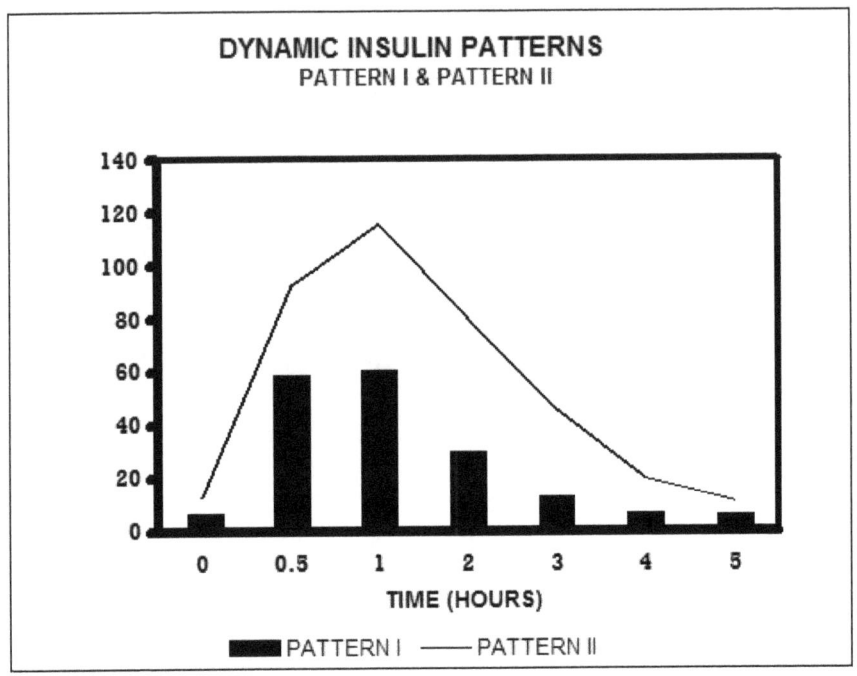

Normal fasting range: 0–30 microunits/ml
½-h or 1-h peak above fasting range
Delayed return to fasting range
2-h + 3-h sum = > 60 microunits/ml

N = 5,138

	F	½-h	1-h	2-h	3-h	4-h	5-h
Mean	13	93	116	80	46	20	11

2-h + 3-h sum = 126 microunits/ml

Pattern II is hyperinsulinemia.

Insulin Pattern II Distribution:
Normal glucose tolerance   4,223 of 9,598   (44%)
Impaired glucose tolerance   749 of 2,775   (27%)
Diabetes mellitus glucose tolerance 166 of 2,011   (8%)

Insulin Pattern II is hyperinsulinemia (insulin resistance), type 2 diabetes. Insulin Pattern II identifies type 2 diabetes not only with the diabetes mellitus glucose tolerance, but also with the impaired glucose tolerance and the normal glucose tolerance.

This dynamic diabetes insulin pattern II demonstrates hyperinsulinemia (increased insulin) by its prominent peaking and its striking delay in returning to the fasting level.

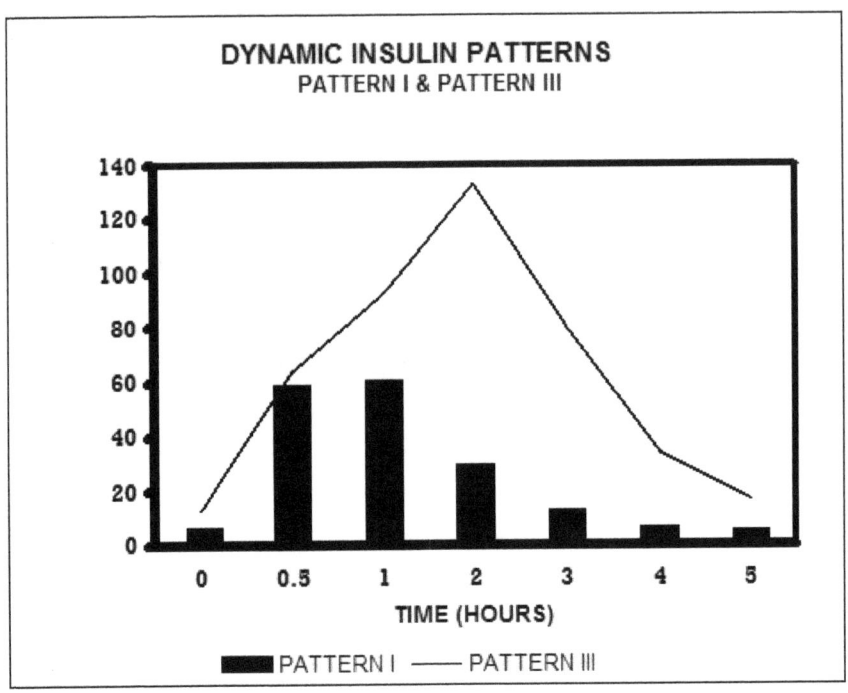

Normal fasting range: 0–30 microunits/ml
Delayed peak 2-h or 3-h
Delayed return to fasting range

N = 5,245

	F	½-h	1-h	2-h	3-h	4-h	5-h
Mean	13	64	93	133	80	34	17

2-h + 3-h sum = 213 microunits/ml

Pattern III is hyperinsulinemia.

Insulin Pattern III Distribution:
Normal glucose tolerance	2,303 of 9,598	(24%)
Impaired glucose tolerance	1,610 of 2,775	(58%)
Diabetes mellitus glucose tolerance	1,332 of 2,011	(66%)

Insulin Pattern III is hyperinsulinemia (insulin resistance), type 2 diabetes. Insulin Pattern III identifies type 2 diabetes not only in diabetes mellitus glucose tolerance but also with the impaired glucose tolerance and the normal glucose tolerance.

This dynamic diabetes insulin pattern III (increased insulin) provides a striking contrast to the normal pattern.

The 2-h — 3-h peaking is overwhelming!

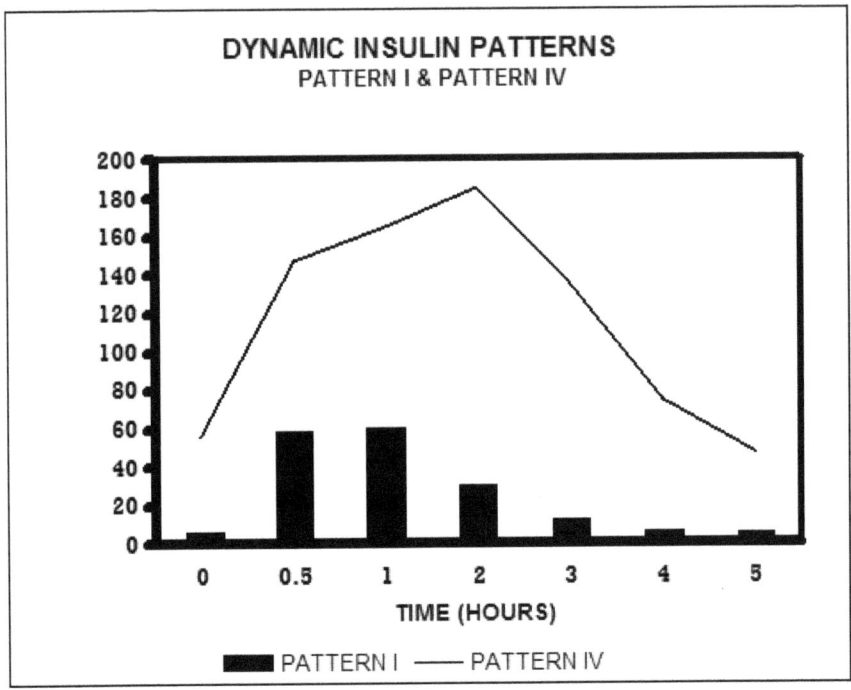

Higher fasting greater than 0–30 microunits/ml
Delayed peak 1-h or 2-h
Delayed return to fasting range

$N \geq 1{,}181$

	F	½-h	1-h	2-h	3-h	4-h	5-h
Mean	56	147	165	185	135	75	47

2-h + 3-h sum ≥320 microunits/ml

Pattern IV is hyperinsulinemia.

Insulin Pattern IV Distribution:
Normal glucose tolerance   576 of 9,598   (6%)
Impaired glucose tolerance   278 or 2,775   (10%)
Diabetes mellitus glucose tolerance 327 of 2,011   (16%)

Insulin Pattern IV is hyperinsulinemia (insulin resistance), type 2 diabetes. Insulin Pattern IV identifies type 2 diabetes not only in the diabetes mellitus glucose tolerance, but also with the impaired glucose tolerance and the normal glucose tolerance.

In Table 2, fasting insulin distribution in 14,384 oral glucose tolerances with insulin assays, 8 percent of fasting insulins greater than 30 microunits/ml identified hyperinsulinemia (insulin resistance), type 2 diabetes. This is insulin Pattern IV. Insulin Pattern IV occurred in 6 percent of the 9,598 normal glucose tolerances, 10 percent of the 2,775 impaired glucose tolerances, and 16 percent of the 2,011 diabetes mellitus glucose tolerances.

Although elevated fasting insulins above normal identify hyperinsulinemia, type 2 diabetes, the sequential (massive) increased insulins as demonstrated in the graph reinforce the diagnosis of type 2 diabetes.

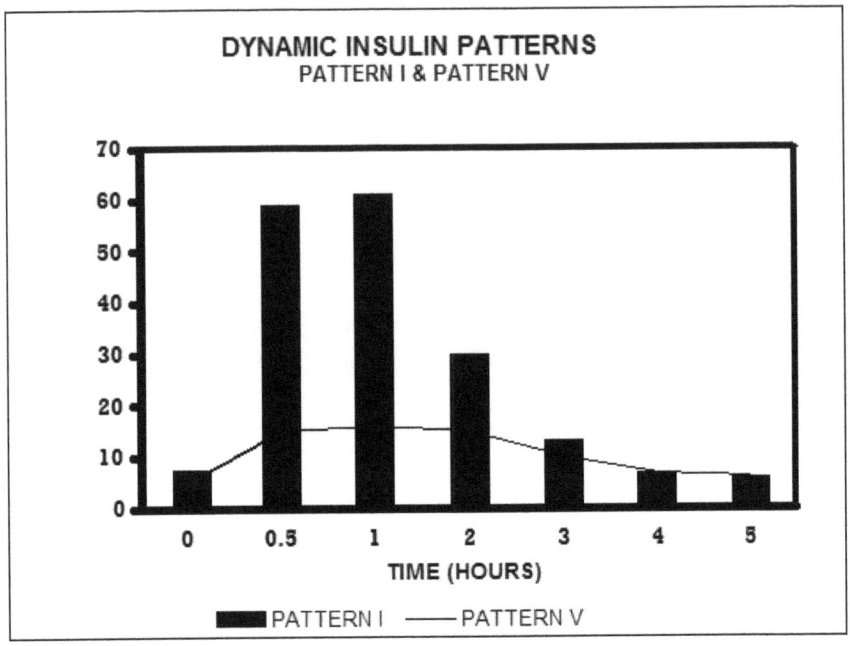

All values within fasting range 0–30 microunits/ml
Low insulin response, hypoinsulinemia

N = 597

	F	1/2-h	1-h	2-h	3-h	4-h	5-h
Mean	5	15	16	15	10	7	6

2-h + 3-h sum = 25 microunits/ml

Pattern V is hypoinsulinemia, low insulin response

Insulin Pattern V Distribution:
Normal glucose tolerance   384 of 9,578   (4%)
Impaired glucose tolerance   55 of 2,775   (2%)
Diabetes mellitus glucose tolerance 158 of 2,011   (8%)

Insulin Pattern V is hypoinsulinemia, the sine qua non of type 1 diabetes. Hypoinsulinemia per se identifies type 1 diabetes with DMGT, IGT, and NGT. Low insulin with high blood sugars (DMGT), type 1 diabetes, hyperglycemia phase is identified. Hypoinsulinemia with IGT and NGT identifies type 1 diabetes in-situ, (occult diabetes), prehyperglcemia.

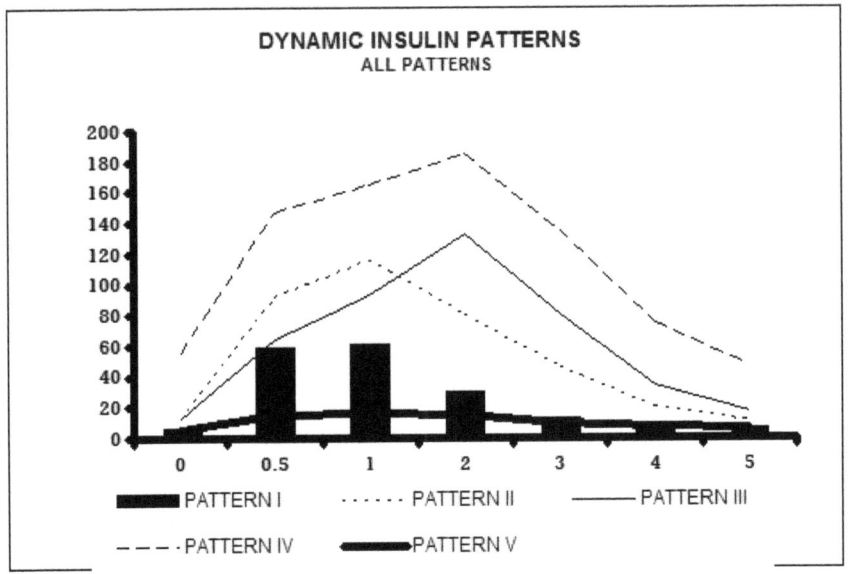

The above graphic is the illustration of Table 3 (page 43). Mean Insulin Values, Microunits/ml in 14,384 Oral Glucose Tolerances.

Increased Insulin (Hyperinsulinemia)

Is

Type 2 Diabetes

Decreased Insulin (Hypoinsulinemia)

Is

Type 1 Diabetes

Table 3. Mean Insulin Values, Microunits/ml in 14,384 Oral Glucose Tolerances

Pattern	Fasting	½ h	1 h	2 h	3 h	4 h	5 h
I (n=2223)							
	8	59	61	30	13	7	6
SE	0.1	0.8	1.0	0.2	0.2	0.1	0.2
II (n=5138)							
	13	93	116	80	46	20	11
SE	0.1	0.9	1.1	0.9	0.7	0.4	0.2
III (n=5245)							
	13	64	93	133	80	34	17
SE	0.2	0.7	1.0	1.4	1.0	0.6	0.4
IV (n=1181)							
	56	147	165	185	135	75	47
SE	3.8	5.5	5.6	5.7	6.1	6.7	8.9
V (n=597)							
	5	15	16	15	10	7	6
SE	0.2	0.3	0.3	0.3	0.3	0.3	0.2

Pattern I = euinsulin, normal, nondiabetes with NGT and IGT
Type 1 diabetes, potential with DMGT

Patterns II, III, IV = hyperinsulin, type 2 diabetes with DMGT, IGT, and NGT

Pattern V = hypoinsulin is type 1 diabetes with DMGT, IGT and NGT.
With IGT and NGT type 1 diabetes is in-situ (occult type 1 diabetes), prehyperglycemia.

References:
1. Kraft, J. R. 1974. "Glucose/insulin tolerance: A routine clinical laboratory tool enhancing diabetes detection." In O. B. Hunter, ed. *Radioassay: Clinical Concepts*. (Skokie, Illinois: G. D. Searle), 91–106.
2. Kraft, J. R. 1975. Detection of diabetes mellitus in-situ (occult diabetes). *Lab Med* 6(2):10–22.
3. Kraft, J. R. 1983. "Insulin and Glucagon." In B. Rothfeld, ed. *Nuclear Medicine in Vitro*. 2nd ed. Philadelphia: J. B. Lippincott), 211–23.
4. Kraft J. R. 1988. "Insulin assay diabetic state identification, a specific diagnostic tool for the noninsulin-dependent diabetic state, a metabolic disorder." In C. F. Claussen, M. V. Kirtane, and K. Schlitter, eds. *Vertigo, Nausea, Tinnitus, and Hypoacusia in Metabolic Disorders*. (Amsterdam: Elsevier), 503–06.
5. Kraft, J. R. 1997. IMx (Abbott) Immunoassay of Insulin: A Practical Alternative to RIA Hyperinsulinemia Identification in Idiopathic Neurootology and Other Hyperinsulin Metabolic Disorders. *Int Tinnitus J* 3(2):13–16.
6. Kraft, J. R. 1998. Hyperinsulinemia: Merging history with idiopathic tinnitus, vertigo, and hearing loss. *Int Tinnitus J* 4(2):1–4.

13

THE ORAL GLUCOSE TOLERANCE: 1918–2007

THE 100-G 3-H sugar tolerance test presented by Janney and Isaacson (1918) was primarily intended for the evaluation and diagnosis of endocrine disorders and only secondarily for diabetes. This was the forerunner of the standard 3-h 100-g oral glucose tolerance test.

Todd (*Clinical Diagnosis and Laboratory Methods*, Fifth Edition, 1925) modified the test to include a ½-h with the fasting and the 1-h, 2-h, and 3-h blood sugar specimens. The results were then plotted on a graph of blood sugar curves. Todd had cited that in healthy persons, blood taken in the morning before breakfast contained about 100 mg of sugar (dextrose) per 100 cc with 90–120 mg being widely accepted as the upper and lower normal limits, with higher values constituting hyperglycemia. The blood sugar curves were greatly prolonged in diabetes. This information was considered superfluous when the fasting levels revealed pronounced hyperglycemia. In mild hyperglycemia, however, the test was found most useful. Todd had emphasized that the test had great value in the early diagnosis of diabetes and even the "prediabetic state."

Standardization of the oral glucose tolerance test (Report of the Committee on Statistics of the American Diabetes Association 1969. *Diabetes* 18:299) provided the Wilkerson Point System guidelines for 100-g oral glucose tolerance interpretation.

In 1979, the National Diabetes Data Group (*Diabetes* 128:1039–57) provided a classification of diabetes mellitus and other categories of glucose intolerance. The 100-g glucose load which had been in place since 1925 was now 75 g. Where the 50-g glucose load had prevailed in Europe and the 100-g load in the U. S., the compromise of a 75-g load was agreed upon. It was the consensus that glucose tolerance values with a 75-g load were relatively equivalent. The normal fasting blood glucose was now to be less than 115 mg/dl. The 100-g glucose load was retained for gestational diabetes mellitus testing and is still the recommended standard (American Diabetes Association Clinical Practice Recommendations. 2007. *Diabetes Care*, Suppl 1).

In 1979, we had 5,000+ oral glucose tolerance tests with insulin assay, all with the standard 100-g glucose load. Insulin assay patterns of euinsulinemia, hyperinsulinemia, and hypoinsulinemia had been established. The medical staff requested that we keep the 100-g dose for adults and for gestational diabetes testing. It was further requested that the 75-g oral dose and/or equivalent be for children and/or others under 20 years of age. The medical staff's requests were complied with. We had 651 in the 14–20 year age group and 113 in the 3–13 year age group who received the 75-g load or equivalent. The insulin assay patterns with the 75-g load were equally applicable to the 100-g glucose load.

In 1997, the American Diabetes Association issued new diagnostic and classification criteria:

- Fasting blood glucose (FBG) lowered to less than 110 mg/dl.
- FBG ≥126 mg/dl classified as probably diabetes mellitus to be confirmed by subsequent examinations.
- Juvenile diabetes now to be called type 1 diabetes.
- Adult-onset diabetes now to be called type 2 diabetes.

These changes were long overdue. Both types could and did occur in any age group.

Type 1 diabetes is an insulin deficiency producing the classic symptoms of polyuria, polydipsia, and weight loss with polyphagia—leading to ketoacidosis, coma, and death. The Egyptians described this condition, and it still occurs today. Type 1 diabetes is estimated to be 5 percent of the diabetes population worldwide. The onset can be abrupt, presenting with ketoacidosis and marked hyperglycemia. Type 1 diabetes is seen most frequently in children and adolescents.

Type 2 diabetes affects 95 percent of the diabetic population, and is insidious in onset. Hyperglycemia is a late manifestation of type 2 diabetes. The insidiousness of type 2 diabetes is best illustrated by the estimated 40+ million undiagnosed people in this country who don't know that they have it and, for the most part, don't care. You, the reader, may be one of them. Except for being overweight or obese, many, but not all, consider themselves to be in good health.

In 2006, the Expert Committee (ADA) confirmed their previous views that there is an intermediate group of subjects whose glucose levels are short of meeting ADA criteria for diabetes but were too high to be considered nor-

mal. (American Diabetes Association, Clinical Practice Recommendations, Suppl 1, 2006):
- FBG less than 100 mg/dl = normal fasting glucose
- FBG 100–125 mg/dl = impaired fasting glucose (IFG)
- FBG greater than 126 mg/dl = provisional diagnosis of diabetes.

75-g oral glucose tolerance:
- 2-h postload glucose less than 140 mg/dl = normal glucose tolerance (NGT)
- 2-h postload glucose 140–199 mg/dl = impaired glucose tolerance (IGT)
- 2-h postload glucose greater than 200 mg/dl = provisional diagnosis of diabetes.

The 14,384 oral glucose tolerances distributed into age groups identified diabetes mellitus glucose tolerances (DMGT 2,011), impaired glucose tolerances (IGT 2,775), and normal glucose tolerances (NGT 9,598) by American Diabetes Association oral glucose tolerance standards (2006).

The insulin assay with the 14,384 oral glucose tolerances further identified hyperinsulinemia (insulin resistance) type 2 diabetes—not only in the DMGT but also in the IGT and NGT. In addition, insulin assay identified nondiabetes in the IGT and the NGT.

The awesome shortcomings of the oral glucose tolerance per se *without* the insulin assays are demonstrated in each age category. The importance of hyperinsulinemia/insulin resistance identification is that the pathology occurrence of type 2 diabetes is not only in those with DMGT, but also occurs in those with IGT and NGT.

Table 4. Fasting Blood Glucose in 14,384 Oral Glucose Tolerance Test with Insulin Assays Designated Normal Glucose Tolerance (NGT), Impaired Glucose Tolerance (IGT), and Diabetes Mellitus Glucose Tolerance (DMGT).

Insulin Patterns	I‡	II$	III	IV	V¶
	(N=2223)	(N=5138)	(N=5245)	N=1181	(N=597)
DMGT	118 ± 71†	126 ± 45	125 ± 45	140 ± 54	240 ± 100
(N=2011)	28	166	1332	327	158
IGT	96 ± 14	97 ± 14	97 ± 14	102 ± 13	102 ± 16
(N=2775)	83	749	1610	278	55
NGT	86 ± 11	85 ± 11	85 ± 11	89 ± 12	84 ± 11
(N=9598)	2112	4223	2303	576	384

* To convert the fasting blood glucose to millimoles per liter, multiply by 0.05551.
† The plus-minus values are means ± standard deviation.
‡ The insulin Pattern I is euinsulinemia. When associated with normal or impaired glucose tolerance, the euinsulinemia designated normal/nondiabetic. When associated with diabetes mellitus glucose tolerance, it designated relative insulin deficiency, type 1 diabetes, potential.
$ Insulin patterns II, III, and IV designated hyperinsulinemia, insulin resistance, type 2 diabetes.
¶ Insulin Pattern V with all values below fasting range (30 micro units per milliliter) designates hypoinsulinemia. When associated with DMGT, IGT and NGT, type 1 diabetes is identified. Type 1 diabetes with IGT and NGT is type 1 diabetes in-situ (occult type 1 diabetes), prehyperglycemia.

14

PATHOLOGY OF TYPE 2 DIABETES

Hyperinsulinemia (insulin resistance)
(NGT – IGT – DMGT)
|
Endothelial Dysfunction
|
Vascular Pathology Dissemination
|
Macroangiopathy – Microangiopathy (Atherosclerosis)
|
Coronary Artery Disease
|
Cerebral Vascular Disease
|
Nephropathy
|
Peripheral Vascular Disease
|
Gestational Diabetes

Pathology of Hyperinsulinemia ⇔ Pathology of Type 2 Diabetes

Robert W. Stout, MD, FRCP, Professor of Geriatric Medicine at Queen's University of Belfast, Northern Ireland, addressed the relationship of insulin to atherosclerosis in diabetes. Professor Stout's investigation, research, and review of the literature concluded that, "The arterial wall is an insulin sensitive tissue. Animal experimentation showed that chronic exposure to high concentrations of insulin resulted in the development of lipid-filled lesions similar to those of early atherosclerosis. Thus, insulin has the ability to promote changes in the artery, which in the long term, may progress to atherosclerosis." (The relationship of abnormal circulating insulin levels to atherosclerosis. 1977. *Atherosclerosis* 27:1–13.) Dr. Stout further concluded that, "Vascular disease is one of the commonest, as well as one of the most serious chronic complications of diabetes. Diabetics are susceptible to disease of both the large muscular arteries, particularly those supplying the myocardium, the brain and the lower limbs and the capillaries of which those of the retina and the glomerulus are the most important clinically." (Diseases and atherosclerosis—The role of insulin. *Diabetologia* 16(1979): 141–50.) In conclusion, Dr. Stout stated the following hypothesis:

The high frequency of atherosclerosis and its complications in the presence of hyperglycemia and diabetes is now well established. The risk of hyperglycemia is associated with the arterial disease itself, as well as with its complications. While the presence of hyperlipidemia or hypertension may occur with the development of the vascular disease, epidemiological studies indicate there is an additional factor associated with diabetes itself.

There is little evidence that hyperglycemia directly contributes to the development of atherosclerosis. The generally reported lack of relationship between the severity of diabetes and the vascular complications... suggest that hyperglycemia is not the factor linking diabetes with atherosclerosis. The possibility that insulin contributes to the development of the large vessel complications of diabetes has been explored, and evidence has been presented that insulin stimulates arterial smooth muscle cell proliferation and lipid synthesis in the arterial wall.

> —"Diabetes and atherosclerosis." In J. S. Bajaj, ed. *Insulin and Metabolism*. Amsterdam, London, New York: Excerpta Medica 27(1979): 1–13.

Dr. Stout's investigations of the 1970s—that insulin, particularly increased insulin (hyperinsulinemia), produced an effect on arterial vessels including capillaries—have now been identified with the endothelium of the arterial vessels and called *endothelial dysfunction*. The endothelium is the innermost single layer of cells lining capillaries and all arterial vessels. The distribution of capillaries throughout the body accounts for the microangiopathy of the retina of the eye, the glomeruli of the kidney, the interstitial myocardium of the heart, and the neurootology of the central nervous system.

Diabetes Epidemic and You / JOSEPH R. KRAFT MD

The pathology of diabetes mellitus is vascular. This includes all major arteries, all minor arteries, and all capillaries. All are lined by a thin epithelium called endothelium. By this widespread arterial distribution, every organ has a potential for pathology.

There is one specific lesion upon light-microscopy examination definitive for diabetes mellitus. *It is intracapillary glomerulosclerosis of the kidney.* This microscopic finding, which is also a clinical entity, was described by Kimmelstiel and Wilson as a specific pathology of the kidney in diabetes mellitus. This occurs in type 2 diabetes of long duration.

It must be noted that type 1 diabetics, all of whom receive exogenous insulin over their lifetime, are thereby made hyperinsulinemic. As a consequence, the pathology of type 1 diabetes now becomes indistinguishable from the hyperinsulinemic (insulin resistant) pathology of type 2 diabetes.

Autopsy examinations of the pancreas gland in known diabetics have not revealed specific findings. Amyloid has received the most attention, but is also found in nondiabetics. As a pathologist with a cumulative autopsy experience of over 3,000+ postmortem examinations, atherosclerosis, focal or diffuse, was a finding in every person over 40 years of age, men and women. In coroner cases, traumatic deaths of individuals under 40 years of age, findings of atherosclerosis were not uncommon. The youngest was an 18-year-old male, whose autopsy revealed incidental findings of atheroma-arteriosclerosis. A surprise to many was the presence of atheroma-atherosclerosis in the young soldiers of the Korean War as reported by the Armed Forces Institute of Pathology. With the exception of the specific lesion of intracapillary glomerulosclerosis of the kidney, diabetes mellitus is not an autopsy diagnosis. *This is due to the failure of acknowledgement that atheroma-atherosclerosis is the primary pathology of diabetes mellitus.*

Cardiovascular disease complications are the leading cause of morbidity and mortality in people with diabetes. Diabetes increases the development of cardiovascular disease up to fivefold. As many as 80 percent of patients with type 2 diabetes die from cardiovascular complications. Cardiovascular disease in diabetes mellitus consists mainly of coronary artery disease with or without infarction, congestive heart failure, and idiopathic cardiomyopathy. Diabetes, the most common endocrine disorder, had an estimated global prevalence of 140 million adults in 1997. (H. King, R. E. Aubert, and W. H. Herman, Global burden of diabetes, 1995–2025: Prevalence, numerical estimates and projections. *CVD Pre* 21(1998): 1414–31.) In the world population, there are millions of undiagnosed prediabetics with normal fasting or impaired fasting blood glucoses. Please see Table 1, Chapter 2: Fasting Blood Glucose—What is Normal?

A brief review:
- 40 percent of the 2,011 diabetes mellitus glucose tolerances (DMGT) had fasting blood glucoses less than 110 mg/dl, of which 20 percent were less than 100 mg/dl.
- The individuals with normal fasting blood glucose may indeed be quite comfortable that they are nondiabetic—that is until they have their first heart attack.

The number of individuals who were not identified as diabetic until after their heart attack is legion. The *Blaylock Wellness Report*, the NewsMax monthly newsletter (January 2007), states, "Heart attacks kill nearly a million Americans a year—rich and poor, the famous and the forgotten. Cardiovascular disease is so common that 64 million Americans suffer some form of it (and 34 million of these folks are age 65 or younger)." Cardiac deaths are the leading cause of death in the U. S. of which diabetes is the number one contributor. *Those with cardiovascular disease not identified with diabetes are simply undiagnosed.*

Dr. Stout in 1977 identified the origin of the pathology of type 2 diabetes as vascular (arterial), directly related to hyperinsulinemia and not to hyperglycemia. The pathology of type 2 diabetes as outlined is mainly the following:

1. Cardiovascular disease
    a. Coronary artery disease
    b. Congestive heart failure
    c. Idiopathic cardiomyopathy
    d. Coronary microvascular dysfunction
2. Cerebral vascular disease
    a. Stroke—kills over 160,000 a year in the U. S. and often without warning
    b. Transient ischemic attack (TIA)
3. Nephropathy
    a. Hypertension
    b. Nephrosclerosis—arterial and arteriolar
4. Retinopathy—major cause of blindness among adults aged 20-74 years
5. Neuropathy
    a. Autonomic—cardiovascular
    b. Peripheral—distal symmetric polyneuritis
    c. Central—neurootological
6. Peripheral arterial disease
7. Penile erectile dysfunction
8. Gestational Diabetes

9. Peyronie's Disease, penile arteriosclerosis of the corpora cavernosa with erectile curvature

Pathology of type 2 diabetes ⇔ Pathology of hyperinsulinemia

Up to 21 percent of patients with type 2 diabetes have retinopathy at the time of their first diagnosis of diabetes. (B. S. Fong, L. Aiello, T. W. Gardener, G. L. King, G. Blankenship, et al. 2003. Diabetes retinopathy. *Diabetes Care* 26, Suppl 1.) Recent data shows that retinopathy (blood vessel changes in the retina of the eye) begins to develop at least seven years before the clinical diagnosis of type 2 diabetes.

The onset of type 2 diabetes probably occurs at least 12 years before the clinical diagnosis. (Harris, M. I. 1993. Undiagnosed NIDDM: Clinical and public health issues. *Diabetes Care* 16:642–52.)

In 1972, Siperstein and associates reported electron-microscopic findings of basement membrane hypertrophy (thickening of the endothelium of renal glomeruli) present in 98.6 percent of 51 overt diabetic patients. This was 50 of 51, with the one being at the upper limit of their normal. They had noted that this finding of diabetic microangiopathy *preceded* the manifestation of diabetes mellitus by months or years. Even more remarkable was their finding that 50 percent of genetic prediabetics tested demonstrated basement membrane hypertrophy *prior* to the onset of detectable carbohydrate abnormalities. Their "genetic" prediabetics were those whose parents were diabetics. This important basic impact of the Siperstein group—finding definitive histopathology by electron microscopy prior to detectable carbohydrate abnormalities—went unrecognized. (Siperstein, M. S., R. H. Unger, and L. L. Madison. "Further Electron Microscopic Studies of Diabetic Microangiopathy." In R. H. Camerini-Davalos and H. S. Cole, eds. *Early Diabetes: Advances in Metabolic Disorders*, Suppl 1. (New York: Academic Press, 1972), 261–71. Worldwide medicine at the time of Siperstein and even today is still harnessed to the identification of diabetes and prediabetes mainly by the fasting blood glucose. (American Diabetes Association Clinical Practice Recommendations, *Diabetes Care* 30 (2007) Suppl 1.)

Additional References:
1. Jarret, R. J. 1988. Is insulin atherogenic? *Diabetologia* 31:71–5.
2. Steinberg, H. O., H. Chaker, R. Leaming, A. Johnson, G. Brechtel, and A. Baron. 1996. Obesity/insulin resistance is associated with endothelial dysfunction. Implications for the syndrome of insulin resistance." *J Clin Invest* 97(11):2601–10.

15

Hyperinsulinemia: Clinical Pathology

THE FIRST MAJOR impact of hyperinsulinemia in the clinical arena was in the discipline of neurootology. In 1977, Updegraff identified hyperinsulinemia with idiopathic Ménière's disease. His cases were an intermix of normal, impaired, and diabetes mellitus glucose tolerances with insulin assays. All revealed hyperinsulinemia of type 2 diabetes. Under the guidance of skilled nutritionists, all who had maintained nutritional compliance experienced sustained clinical response.

Updegraff's studies were substantiated by others: Mangabeira-Albernaz and Fukuda (1984), Proctor and Proctor (1988), and Fukuda, Juliane, and Mangabeira-Albernaz (1988). In addition, Proctor and Proctor (1988) independently identified hyperinsulinemia as the major diagnostic factor in their cases of idiopathic dizziness and tinnitus. Studies by D'Avila and Lavinsky (2005) and additional studies by Zuma e Maia and Lavinsky (2006) show that hyperinsulinemia is one of the most frequent causes of cochleovestibular syndromes.

The clinical pathology of hyperinsulinemia type 2 diabetes associated with euglycemic glucose tolerances has been identified as an etiologic factor in atherosclerosis—mainly coronary artery disease, essential hypertension, primordial follicle dysfunction, gestational diabetes, and idiopathic peripheral neuropathy—in addition to the pioneer identification of idiopathic headache (Ménière's), tinnitus, vertigo, and hearing loss. A clinical pathology of hyperinsulinemia for which little attention has been given is functional hypoglycemia, which is being addressed in Chapter 16.

References:
1. Updegraff, W. R. 1977. Impaired carbohydrate metabolism in idiopathic Ménière's disease. *Ear, Nose, Throat J* 56:60–63.
2. Updegraff, W. R. "A new metabolic approach to headache and dizziness." In E. Meyers, ed. *New Dimensions in Otorhinolaryngology—Head and Neck Surgery*, Vol. 2 (Elsevier Science Publishers, B. V.) 1985, The Netherlands
3. Updegraff, W. R. "The relationship of vertigo/headache to atherosclerosis." In C. F. Claussen and M. V. Kirtane, eds. *Vertigo, nausea, tinnitus and hearing loss in cardiovascular diseases.* (The Netherlands: Elsevier Science Publishers B. V.), 1986.
4. Updegraff, W. R. "Ménière's, migraine and general medicine." In C. F. Clausen, M. V. Kirtane, and K. Schlitter, eds. *Vertigo, nausea, tinnitus and hypoacusia in metabolic disorders.* (The Netherlands: Elsevier Science Publishers B. V.), 1988.
5. Mangabeira-Albernaz, P. L., and Y. Fukuda. 1984. Glucose, insulin and the inner ear pathology. *Acta Otolaringol*, 496–501.
6. Fukuda, Y., L. Juliane, and P. L. Mangabeira-Albernaz. "The physiopathological influence of hyperinsulinemia on the origin of Ménière's disease." In C. F. Claussen, M. V. Kirtane, and K. Schlitter, eds. *Vertigo, nausea, tinnitus, and hypoacusia in metabolic disorders.* (Amsterdam: Elsevier), 1988, 379–83.
7. Proctor, C. A., and T. D. Proctor. "Hyperinsulinemia and tinnitus." In C. F. Claussen, M. V. Kirtane and K. Schlitter, eds. *Vertigo, nausea, tinnitus and hypoacusia in metabolic disorders* (Amsterdam: Elsevier), 1988, 255–57.
8. D'Avila, C., and L. Lavinsky. 2005. Glucose and insulin profiles and their correlation in Ménière's disease. *Int Tinnitus J* 11:170–76.
9. Zuma e Maia, F. C. and L. Lavinsky 2006. Distortion product otoacoustic emissions in an animal model of induced hyperinsulinemia. *Int Tinnitus J* 12:133–39.
10. Ganaca, M. M., H. H. Caovilla, F. F. Ganaca, and G. Serafini. 1995. Dietary management for tinnitus control with hyperinsulinemia—a retrospective study. *Int Tinnitus J* 1:41–5.
11. Kraft, J. R. 1995. Hyperinsulinemia (insulin resistance)—the common denominator of subjective idiopathic tinnitus and other peripheral neurootological disorders. *Int Tinnitus J* 1:46–53.
12. Zarvaroni, I., E. Bonora, M. Pagliara, et al., 1989. Risk factor for coronary artery disease in healthy persons with hyperinsulinemia and normal glucose tolerance. *N Engl J Med* 320:702–06.

13. Ferrannini, E., G. Buzzigoli, R. Bonadonna, et al. 1987. Insulin resistance in essential hypertension. *N Engl J Med* 317:350–57.
14. Reaven, G. M., and B. B. Hoffman, 1987. A role for insulin in the etiology and course of hypertension? *Lancet* 2:435–37.
15. Perez-Pelaez, M., R. S. Jeyendran, J. R. Kraft, and K. T. Sie. "Abnormal insulin pattern and its relationship to defective folliculogenisis in infertile patients". Abstract in T. E. Soon, S. S. Ratman and L. S. Min, eds. *Proceedings 12th World Congress on Fertility and Sterility* (Singapore: Gyne Soc of Singapore 4:1094, 1986).
16. Kraft, J. R. "Hyperinsulinemia /Insulin Resistance, the New Gold Standard of Gestational Diabetes Diagnosis, a Distinct Clinical Entity." Rudolph Holmes Memorial Lecture. Chicago Gync Soc, February 16, 1990.

16

FUNCTIONAL HYPOGLYCEMIA: CLINICAL FACT OR FICTION?

ON JUNE 6, 1993, I presented a paper at the XXI Proceedings of the NES in Linköping, Sweden, entitled "Functional hypoglycemia: clinical fact or fiction, classification by glucose/insulin tolerance." My presentation time was 2:00 p.m., after the noonday lunch. I started my presentation, acknowledging a difference of opinion as to whether or not this subject— also known as *postprandial drop*—was a clinical condition. I asked the audience to observe those sitting next to them. Over half of the audience was already dozing into dream world. The half that was still alert became believers.

In our 14,384 oral glucose tolerances with insulin assays, there were 5,128 or 36 percent with lowered glucose levels after the first hour of peaking. The glucose levels were between 20 and 59 mg/dl. The 5,128 glucoses were in one of the following levels:

        20–30 mg/dl   (2%)
        31–40 mg/dl   (10%)
        41–50 mg/dl   (35%)
        51–59 mg/dl   (53%)

Seventy-five percent or over 3,858 of the 5,128 were hyperinsulinemia, type 2 diabetes.

    DMGT (diabetes mellitus glucose tolerance)
        196 with hypoglycemia:
        193   or 98% hyperinsulinemia, type 2 diabetes
        3   or 2% hypoinsulinemia, type 1 diabetes, potential, alimentary hypoglycemia, postprandial

IGT (impaired glucose tolerance)
>   492 with hypoglycemia:
>   - 427 or 97% hyperinsulinemia, type 2 diabetes
>   - 15 or 3% euinsulin, nondiabetes, alimentary hypoglycemia, postprandial

NDGT (nondiagnostic glucose tolerance)
>   716 with hypoglycemia:
>   - 638 or 89% hyperinsulinemia, type 2 diabetes
>   - 78 or 11% euinsulinemia, nondiabetes, alimentary hypoglycemia, postprandial

NGT (normal glucose tolerance)
>   3,724 with hypoglycemia:
>   - 2,532 or 68% hyperinsulinemia, type 2 diabetes
>   - 1,192 or 32% euinsulinemia, nondiabetes, alimentary hypoglycemia, postprandial

Conclusions:
1. In 5,128 glucose/insulin tolerances with hypoglycemia, 75 percent (3,858) demonstrated hyperinsulinemia, type 2 diabetes.
2. Hypoglycemia associated with hyperinsulinemia, type 2 diabetes is designated *functional hypoglycemia*.
3. Functional hypoglycemia is identified by insulin assay with oral glucose tolerance whenever the lowered glucose levels are between 20 and 50 ml/dl after the second hour up to the fourth hour postglucose load.
4. *Alimentary hypoglycemia* is characterized by glucose/insulin tolerance with euinsulinemia or hypoinsulinemia. The lowered glucose levels in hypoglycemic range occur before the two-hour postglucose load.
5. The hypoglycemia designated alimentary is due to rapid gastric emptying or "dumping." This occurs with gastric resection, duodenal pathology, or a functional evacuation by accelerated peristalsis of varied causes.
6. *Postprandial hypoglycemia* joins obesity as an indicator for the identification or exclusion of hyperinsulinemia, type 2 diabetes by oral glucose tolerance with insulin assay.

In the real world, postprandial hypoglycemia, whether functional or alimentary, is truly a subjective clinical entity. This can best be expressed by the cartoon "Broom-Hilda" by R. Myers in the *Chicago Tribune*, April 26, 1976. This gifted cartoonist presents four sequential drawings. The first introduced a silent Broom-Hilda. The second shows her quivering, saying, "Oh Drat!" In the third drawing, she has now quivered down to one-third of her size. In the fourth drawing, she is now totally collapsed, stating, "I hate those sudden drops in blood sugar levels."

I can personally relate to postprandial drop and the clinical hypoglycemic drop during my oral glucose tolerances. The drowsiness lasts about 30 minutes. Reading during this time is almost impossible. Driving an auto is actually dangerous at this time.

I am convinced that hypoglycemia postprandial and hypoglycemia associated with oral glucose tolerance are fact and not fiction.

In the *Wall Street Journal's* September 12, 2008 front-page article entitled "Pilot Fatigue Spurs Calls for New Safeguards," the National Transportation Safety Board is addressing pilot fatigue and the dangers associated with "exhausted, overworked, and downright sleepy pilots." One symptom of fatigue that is being studied is *micro sleep*. What is not being addressed is postprandial drop, the drowsiness following eating. *Postprandial drop* definitely occurs in some of the pilots of commercial airlines. How do I know? Pilots are human; they are not exempt from alimentary or functional lowering of their blood sugars.

Should every pilot, even those with normal blood sugars, be tested by oral glucose tolerance with insulin assays, in order to exclude or identify increased insulins with lowered blood sugars?

ABSOLUTELY NOT!
ONLY THOSE CONCERNED ABOUT THEIR FUTURE!

Reference:

Kraft, J. R. and K. T. Sie. "Functional Hypoglycemia: Clinical Fact or Fiction. Classification by Glucose/Insulin Tolerance, Hyperinsulinemia Identification." In C. F. Clausen, M. V. Kirtane, and D. Schneider, eds. Proceedings of the NES, Volume XXI. Presented June 2–6, 1993 in Linköping, Sweden (Hamburg: Werner Rudat & Co., 1995), 309–11.

17

GESTATIONAL DIABETES

A LANDMARK IN prospective medicine was initiated by the publication of "Criteria for the oral glucose tolerance test in pregnancy" by J. B. O'Sullivan and C. M. Mahan, *Diabetes* 13:278, 1964. It was known that infants with birth weights greater than nine pounds had a higher incidence of maternal and fetal complications. The large infant was a frequent occurrence in those with diabetes. The author applied the standard 100-g oral glucose tolerance test in pregnancy to determine the presence or absence of diabetes. They not only identified those already with diabetes at the onset of the pregnancy, but unveiled a startling finding of the development of diabetes during the pregnancy. This development identified by the oral glucose tolerance became designated Gestational Diabetes Mellitus (GDM). They also observed that most but not all returned to "normal" after the pregnancy was completed, but raised the question of future development of diabetes. This was also a concern of the American Diabetes Association (ADA).

The ADA has recommended that women with GDM should be screened for diabetes six to twelve weeks postpartum. They should be followed up with subsequent screening for the development of diabetes or prediabetes in the years to come. The ADA has further recommended that even those individuals not diagnosed as GDM but who had delivered a baby of nine pounds or more should also have subsequent screening in the years to come.

In our database, there were 374 persons with glucose/insulin tolerances of less than three days postpartum. Two hundred had infant birth weights of nine pounds or more, and 174 had birth weights between eight and nine pounds. Glucose tolerances during their pregnancies are unknown.

NGT = 289
        105 euinsulin, nondiabetes
        38 birth weight ≥8 pounds
        67 birth weight ≥9 pounds

184 hyperinsulin (insulin resistance) type 2 diabetes
   68 birth weight ≥8 pounds
   116 birth weight ≥9 pounds

IGT = 75

3 euinsulin, nondiabetes
   3 birth weight ≥8 pounds
   0 birth weight ≥9 pounds
72 hyperinsulin (insulin resistance) type 2 diabetes
   59 birth weight ≥8 pounds
   16 birth weight ≥9 pound

DMGT = 10 (diabetes mellitus glucose tolerance)

0 euinsulin
9 hyperinsulin (insulin resistance) type 2 diabetes
   8 birth weight ≥8 pounds
   1 birth weight ≥9 pounds
1 hypoinsulin type 1 diabetes, potential
   Birth weight ≥8 pounds

The ADA criteria for GDM are by hyperglycemia glucose values only. The criteria per se fail to identify GDM in those with normal (NGT) or impaired glucose tolerance (IGT). Infants large for gestational age or greater than nine pounds do occur with NGT or IGT during pregnancy. The ADA is aware of this occurrence. It has urged that even though GDM was not diagnosed, that the mother and child be screened for prediabetes and diabetes in the years to come.

Hyperinsulinemia (insulin resistance) is type 2 diabetes, gestational diabetes in pregnancy. In the 374 persons with postpartum oral glucose tolerance with insulin assays, less than three days, the observations of O'Sullivan and Mahan (1964) that many, but not all, with glucose intolerance during pregnancy return to "normal" was concurred. Two hundred of the 374 infants with birth weights greater than nine pounds, and their mothers, became lifetime candidates for prediabetes and diabetes screening.

Also in our database were 131 persons with glucose/insulin tolerance greater than three days up to two years postpartum: Seventy-eight had birth weights equal to or greater than nine pounds, and 53 had birth weights equal to or greater than eight pounds and less than nine pounds.

NGT = 96
- 32 euinsulin, nondiabetes
  - 10 birth weight ≥8 pounds
  - 22 birth weight ≥9 pounds
- 64 hyperinsulin (insulin resistance) type 2 diabetes
  - 24 birth weight ≥8 pounds
  - 40 birth weight ≥9 pounds

IGT = 30
- 8 euinsulin, nondiabetes
  - 6 birth weight ≥8 pounds
  - 2 birth weight ≥9 pounds
- 22 hyperinsulin (insulin resistance) type 2 diabetes
  - 12 birth weight ≥8 pounds
  - 10 birth weight ≥9 pounds

DMGT = 5
- 0 euinsulin
- 5 hyperinsulin (insulin resistance) type 2 diabetes
  - 1 birth weight ≥8 pounds
  - 4 birth weight ≥9 pounds

The 78 infants with birth weights greater than nine pounds, and their mothers, also became lifetime candidates for prediabetes and diabetes screening. This does not mean that those with postpartum euinsulin NGT and euinsulin IGT and birth weights between eight and nine pounds are necessarily free of risk. Should everyone in this category be tested? Of course not! Only those concerned about their future.

Curet, et al. applied insulin assays to the standard 100–g oral glucose tolerance test (OGTT) to 100 persons receiving prenatal care at the University of New Mexico. The tests were performed between 11 and 20 weeks. Ninety-one completed the study. The study was limited to 87 with normal OGTT. The results were the following:
- 18 had normal insulins of which 5 had infants large for gestational age/macrosomia
- 69 had hyperinsulinemia (insulin resistance) type 2 diabetes of which 15 had infants large for gestational age/macrosomia.

Curet concludes that there is a gestational diabetes state characterized by euglycemia with hyperinsulinemia. (Curet, L., Joffe, G., Qualls, C., Kraft, J. 1996.) Plasma insulin secretion during the 3-h glucose tolerance test is a better predictor of perinatal risk than glucose levels. (Abstract. *J Soc Gynecol Investg.* 3 (Suppl 2): A–130.) Dr. Curet, a leader ahead of his time, identified that gestational diabetes is initially characterized by normal glucose tolerance with hyperinsulinemia.

Our data also identified 648 individuals with glucose/insulin tolerance during the 30–36 weeks of pregnancy. They were predominately from the 21–30 year old age group in Part 2.

NGT = 456
        31 euinsulin, nondiabetic
        425 hyperinsulin (insulin resistance) type 2 diabetes of pregnancy (GDM)

IGT = 94
        1 euinsulin, nondiabetic
        93 hyperinsulin (insulin resistance) type 2 diabetes of pregnancy (GDM)

DMGT = 98
        0 euinsulin
        95 hyperinsulin (insulin resistance) type 2 diabetes of pregnancy (GDM)
        3 hypoinsulin, low insulin type 1 diabetes, potential

The oral glucose tolerance (OGT) without insulin assays identified 15 percent or 98 GDM (DMGT) of the 648 persons tested. The OGT with insulin assays identified 613 or 95 percent with GDM, hyperinsulinemia, type 2 diabetes of pregnancy. This included those identified with DMGT and also those with IGT and NGT. In addition, the OGT with insulin assay identified 5 percent that were nondiabetic.

In our testing for GDM during pregnancy, there were 35 persons with two glucose/insulin tolerances.

Initial Examination:

11	First Trimester	(less than 12 weeks)
20	Second Trimester	(13–24 weeks)
4	Third Trimester	(25–36 weeks)

Unchanged from Initial Examination:
4 GDM with hyperinsulinemia type 2 diabetes of pregnancy
11 NGT with hyperinsulinemia, type 2 diabetes of pregnancy

Progression: → Five NGT with hyperinsulinemia to GDN with hyperinsulinemia, type 2 diabetes of pregnancy
→ Two NGT First Trimester to Third Trimester, GDM
→ Three NGT Second Trimester to Third Trimester, GDM

This dynamic transition of normal glucose tolerance with hyperinsulinemia (NGT) to diabetes mellitus glucose tolerance with hyperinsulinemia, type 2 diabetes of pregnancy (GDM) within the short time span of pregnancy is a microcosm of what occurs in nonpregnancy, type 2 diabetes. The transition of NGT to DMGT (GDM) highlights NGT, hyperinsulinemia as the earliest phase of gestational diabetes of pregnancy, type 2 diabetes.

In nonpregnancy, this transition was first identified in 1974. In 1975, it was designated diabetes mellitus in situ (occult diabetes). (Kraft, J. R. 1975. Detection of diabetes mellitus in situ (occult diabetes). *Lab Med* 6, no. 2 (February):10–22.) In nonpregnancy, NGT and IGT to DMGT transition may require many years before the hyperglycemic phase of diabetes becomes manifest.

Progression—second trimester to third trimester:
5 NGT, normal insulin to 5 NGT, hyperinsulinemia type 2 diabetes of pregnancy
1 NGT, normal insulin to IGT, hyperinsulinemia type 2 diabetes of pregnancy
2 NGT, hyperinsulinemia to 2 IGT, hyperinsulinemia type 2 diabetes of pregnancy
1 IGT, hyperinsulinemia to GDM, hyperinsulinemia type 2 diabetes of pregnancy

One again, it is illustrated that hyperinsulinemia is GDM, type 2 diabetes in pregnancy manifested in NGT, IGT, and DMGT.

Regression—second trimester and third trimester:
　3 IGT, hyperinsulinemia, type 2 diabetes of pregnancy
　2 IGT to NGT, hyperinsulinemia type 2 diabetes of pregnancy
　1 IGT to NGT, euinsulin, nondiabetes

The above results illustrate the response of medical management in the second and third trimesters of pregnancy. For information regarding the treatment of gestational diabetes, see K. Ruder, "Friendly Ties." *Diabetes Forecast* (December 2006):55–8.

Gestational diabetes can be treated by improving diet and exercise or with insulin. Just like with type 1 or type 2 diabetes, the goal is to keep blood glucose levels as close to normal as possible during pregnancy to ensure that mother and child are healthy. In most cases, gestational diabetes goes away after birth of the child—but the danger lurks. Twenty to fifty percent of the women who develop gestational diabetes will get type 2 diabetes within the next ten years. What is more, their children have a lifetime risk of obesity and diabetes.

Luckily, there are steps that women with gestational diabetes can take to prevent or delay diabetes. Tips for women who have gestational diabetes:

1. Know where you stand: Get tested for diabetes six weeks after giving birth, and if "normal," get tested at least every three years thereafter.
2. Plan ahead: Talk to your doctor if you plan to get pregnant again and try to get to an ideal weight before you become pregnant.
3. Be active: Exercise for thirty minutes, five times a week. Encourage your kids to be active at least an hour every day.
4. Eat well: Make healthy food choices for the family such as whole grains, fruits and vegetables, fish, lean meats, and low-fat milk and cheese.

— Copyright © 2006 American Diabetes Association From Diabetes Forecast®, December 2006
Reprinted with permission of *The American Diabetes Association*

For information online, go to www.diabetes.org/diabetesforecast or www.diabetes.org/gestational-diabetes.jsp.

Additional References:
1. Kraft, J. R. "Glucose/Insulin Tolerance: A Routine Laboratory Tool Enhancing Diabetes Detection." *Radioassay: Clinical Concepts Symposium on Radioimmunoassay*, Washington, DC, January 28–29, 1974. (Skokie, Illinois: G. D. Searle, 1974:91–106).
2. Kraft, J. R. "The Glucose Tolerance Examination, an Obsolete Procedure." *Symposium on Radioimmunoassay Diagnostic Medicine.* Annual Convention American Medical Association, Chicago, IL, June 26, 1974.
3. Kraft, J. R. Detection of diabetes mellitus in situ (occult diabetes). *Laboratory Medicine* 6, no. 2 (February 1975):10–22.
4. Kraft, J. R. "Hyperinsulinemia/Insulin Resistance—The Proposed New Gold Standard of Gestational Diabetes Diagnosis." Rudolph Holmes Memorial Lecture. Chicago Gynecol Soc, February 16, 1990.
5. Kraft, J. R. "Hyperinsulinemia (Insulin Resistance)—The Diagnostic Identifier of Gestational Diabetes Mellitus." Symposium on Gestational Diabetes. Professor P. A. M. Weise, Director, University of Graz, Austria. 1992.
6. *Diabetes Care* (July 2007): 30 (Suppl 2). http://www.diabetes.org/diabetescare. Proceedings of the Fifth International Workshop-Conference on Gestational Diabetes Mellitus, Chicago, Illinois, November 11–13, 2005.

18

C-Reactive Protein

I AM INCLUDING this review of C-reactive protein (CRP) for your perusal. It has become applicable in relation to heart disease and diabetes.

The C–reactive protein is a laboratory procedure that has now been given a new life. This serum constituent was discovered by interacting the serum of patients who had recovered from pneumococcal infections with C-polysaccharide of that bacterium. Visible flocculates formed, which allowed extensive study and purification of this C-reactive protein of serum in the 1940s.

It was found that CRP is present in serum of patients with disorders other than pneumococcal infections. It rises noticeably whenever there is inflammation with or without tissue necrosis. Many other substances were known to react with CRP, such as nucleotides, various lipids, and other polysaccharides.

The traditional assays for CRP do not have the sensitivity to detect levels required for vascular disease prediction. To alleviate this deficiency, CRP assays of high sensitivity have been developed and are now available.

There has been considerable recent interest in C–reactive protein as a marker of inflammation in cardiovascular disease. The following reference critiques the clinical application of CRP for cardiovascular disease: Ridker, P. M., 2003. Clinical application of C-reactive protein for cardiovascular disease detection and prevention. *Circulation* 107:363.

In multiple prospective studies, it has been reported that the CRP has been of value in predicting myocardial infarction, stroke, peripheral arterial disease, and sudden cardiac death. The CRP levels have also been reported to predict risk of both recurrent ischemia and death among those with stable and unstable angina. In addition, it has been reported to be useful in predicting risk in those undergoing percutaneous angioplasty and especially those presenting with acute coronary syndromes coming to emergency rooms.

Prospective data indicates that the CRP is a better predictor of cardiovascular risk than a low-density lipoprotein (LDL) cholesterol, the standby predictor of cardiovascular disease. The CRP advantage is that "inflammation," (but not the elevated LDL) is associated with the components of the metabolic syndrome. CRP levels are not only demonstrated with "inflammation" of cardiovascular disease, but also with triglycerides, obesity, elevated blood pressure, and elevated fasting blood glucose. In addition, CRP also correlates with endothelial dysfunction, impaired fibrinolysis, and most importantly, insulin resistance, which is hyperinsulinemia, type 2 diabetes. I ask you, the reader, to please note that the clinical conditions associated with CRP, especially its application for cardiovascular disease, is the pathology of insulin resistance, hyperinsulinemia, type 2 diabetes. Please see Chapter 14, Pathology of Type 2 Diabetes.

Inflammation in the prediabetic state is related to increased insulin resistance rather than decreased insulin secretion. (Festa, A. A., J. G. Hanley, R. P. Tracy, R. D'Agostino, and S. M. Haffner. 2003. *Circulation* 108:1822–30.) Their conclusion: "We have shown an increased proinflammatory state in prediabetic individuals (increased CRP) who are predominantly insulin resistant (hyperinsulinemic), but not in those with a primary defect in B-cell function. These results provide additional evidence that prediabetic subjects may be at an increased risk of heart disease, and this risk seems to be restricted to subjects with high insulin resistance (hyperinsulinemia)."

This publication establishes that insulin resistance, hyperinsulinemia per se, gives independent high levels of CRP. Haffner, et al. in "Cardiovascular Risk Factors in Confirmed Prediabetic Individuals" (1990) confirmed my studies of 1975 that prediabetic individuals are hyperinsulinemic.

The association of C- reactive protein with hyperinsulinemia provides an essential dimension to the clinical application of C-reactive protein for cardiovascular disease detection and prevention.

References:
1. Haffner, S. M., M. P. Stern, H. P. Hazuda, B. D. Mitchell, and J. K. Patterson. 1990. Cardiovascular risk factors in confirmed prediabetic individuals. Does the clock for coronary heart disease start ticking before the onset of clinical diabetes? *JAMA* 263, no. 2 (June):2893-98.
2. Kraft, J. R. 1975. Detection of diabetes mellitus in situ (occult diabetes). *Laboratory Medicine* 16, no. 2 (February).

19

Cholesterol: A Risk Factor for Heart Disease and Diabetes?

CHOLESTEROL IS A term for fat-like substances that are in all the body's cells, including blood. Cholesterol is also found in some foods you eat. Your body needs cholesterol to make some hormones and vitamins, and to help digestion. Your body makes all of the cholesterol it needs.

HDL cholesterol or high-density lipoprotein cholesterol is also known as "good" cholesterol. HDL helps to remove cholesterol from your body, so the higher your HDL, the lower your chance of getting heart disease.

LDL cholesterol or low-density lipoprotein cholesterol can lead to a buildup of cholesterol in the arteries and is sometimes called "bad" cholesterol. The higher your LDL level, the greater your risk for heart disease.

Triglycerides are another form of fat in your blood. High triglycerides can raise your risk for heart disease.

All of the above definitions are from the American Diabetes Association's brochure, "Check√Up America—Know your Risk. Lower your Risk for Diabetes and Heart Disease."

The pharmaceutical industry has produced effective medications called *statins*, which lower cholesterol levels. Side effects range from mild to serious; nevertheless, a trillion-dollar industry has blossomed. There is no evidence that cholesterol—by itself—blocks coronary or cerebral arteries, causing heart attacks or strokes. Cholesterol is a co-participant in lipid deposition into the endothelium of arterial vessels damaged by hyperinsulinemia. Please review Chapter 14, Pathology of Type 2 Diabetes.

Heart Check America Coronary Artery Screening Program at the University of Illinois Chicago Medical Center has had many persons with atherosclerotic coronary artery disease in which their cholesterols were normal. I just happen to be one of them. Although asymptomatic, in 1992, I had their Coronary Artery Scanning for Calcification (CASC). It revealed extensive atherosclerosis. My cardiologist interpreted my cardiac thallium stress test as normal. He asked me, in my extensive autopsy experience, had I ever seen a person of my age free of coronary atherosclerosis. My answer was no! In fact, I told him I had never seen one free of atherosclerosis beginning at the age of 40—men or women.

To practice what you preach is a difficult axiom to live by. In 1973, I had my first 100-g oral glucose tolerance with insulin assays. To my surprise, I had an impaired glucose tolerance with hyperinsulinemia. I should not have been surprised, for I was overweight. After three months of nutritional control and intensive exercise, a second examination revealed normal glucose tolerance with euinsulinemia. The weight reduction was rewarding.

Over the next 25 years, I had many glucose/insulin tolerances. They would vary between euglycemia with hyperinsulinemia and euglycemia with euinsulinemia. The variations were directly related to a weight fluctuation of five to ten pounds. My last examination after my retirement was in June 2006. I again was euglycemic with hyperinsulinemia, type 2 diabetes. A most difficult decision for me to make was to be honest with myself. Yes, I am a diabetic! After all, if I tell others that hyperinsulinemia (insulin resistance) is type 2 diabetes and not just "prediabetes," it must also apply to me. I have the coronary atherosclerosis of many years to prove it.

During this last glucose/insulin tolerance (June 2006), between the second and third hours, I experienced a marked postprandial drop. This experience had occurred during my previous examinations whenever hyperinsulinemia was present. Please see Chapter 16 on functional hypoglycemia. In my many years as Director of Laboratories at St. Joseph Hospital in Chicago, Illinois, I had numerous lipid profile examinations. My total cholesterols were less than 160 mg/dl, and the HDL and LDL cholesterols were considered "ideal." On January 9, 2007, my total cholesterol was 142 mg/dl with HDL of 79 mg/dl.

For most people with high cholesterols, prescription medicines are safe and effective. Eating a heart-healthy diet is also safe and effective, and is the very best nonprescription therapy.

20

OVERWEIGHT/OBESE: A RISK FACTOR FOR HEART DISEASE AND DIABETES

OBESITY HAS LONG been recognized as a contributing factor in diabetes mellitus. The Diabetes Data Group, realizing that the definition of obesity is complex and that a satisfactory index of obesity had not been devised, agreed that measures using height and weight—the *Body Mass Index* (BMI)—have the highest correlation with both skin-fold thickness and body density.

$$BMI = Weight (kg) \text{ divided by } Height^2 (m)$$

Furthermore, the BMI has a linear relationship to the index of Percent Desirable Weight (PDW). This is based on medium-frame ideal body weight estimates of The Society of Actuaries. A PDW of 120 percent corresponds to a BMI of 27 for men and 25 for women. National Diabetes Data Group: Classification and diagnosis of diabetes mellitus and other categories of glucose intolerance. (*Diabetes* 28:1039–57 (1979). You will note that the ADA currently defines the healthy range of BMI between 19 and 25. Being skinny is in! However, be careful of anorexia. This is a subclinical mental disorder recognized by others and only rarely, if ever, by the person themselves.

The BMI is not applicable to everyone. Many athletes and non-athletes without an ounce of fat have BMIs labeling them "obese." Table 5, The Obesity and Glucose Tolerance, reveals an obese Chicago population. Among 10,695 persons, it identifies 43 percent as nondiabetic, normal glucose/insulin tolerances and 68 percent of the NIDDM (diabetes mellitus glucose tolerances) as obese.

Table 5. Obesity and Glucose Tolerance

NIH Classification	PDW greater than 120%	Total
IDDM	60%	123
NIDDM	68%	1,313
IGT	62%	1,101
Nondiagnostic	58%	2,076
Normal	46%	6,082
		10,695
Nondiabetic, normal glucose/insulin tolerance	43%	1,628

J. R. Kraft, "Insulin and Glucagon." In B. Rothfeld. *Nuclear Medicine in Vitro*, 2nd ed. (Philadelphia: J. B. Lippincott, 1983), 211–23. Reprinted by permission of Lippincott Williams and Wilkins ©1983.

Insulin resistance, hyperinsulinemia, type 2 diabetes:
  100%   of the 1,313   NIDDM
  95%   of the 1,101   IGT
  88%   of the 2,076   NDGT
  64%   of the 6,082   NGT

Non-obesity is of equal importance. *Not everyone with type 2 diabetes is obese.* Let this not lead you into a false sense of security. Your feelings of security will be further enhanced if your fasting blood sugar is normal. After all, why worry when you feel so good? *Normal weight, normal BMI, normal fasting blood sugar, and normal fasting insulins do not exclude hyperinsulinemia, type 2 diabetes.*

In their January 18, 2007 article entitled "Obesity and Diabetes in the Developing World—A Growing Challenge" in the New England Journal of Medicine, Hossain, Kawar, and El Nakas identify more than 1.1 billion adults worldwide as overweight and 312 million of them as obese. Furthermore, an International Task Force and the World Health Organization revised their definition of obesity for ethnic differences, classifying *1.7 billion children as overweight worldwide.* The authors also noted the worldwide increase of the clinical pathology of type 2 diabetes. No mention was made of the earliest identification of type 2 diabetes with or without obesity.

The relationship of obesity to diabetes with or without normal fasting blood sugars in children and adults mandates the earliest identification of diabetes by the oral glucose tolerance with insulin assays. If YOU are obese—and you know whether you are or not—obesity must be considered hyperinsulin, type 2 diabetes until proven otherwise by oral glucose tolerance with insulin assays. Even if your fasting blood sugar and your cholesterol are "normal," the above applies to YOU. The choice is yours.

21

Know Your Risk Factors for Heart Disease and Diabetes

Cardiometabolic risk factors:
    High cholesterol and lipids (See Chapter 19)
    Overweight/obesity (See Chapter 20)
    Physical inactivity
    High blood pressure
    High blood glucose
    Smoking

    Check√Up America ~ American Diabetes Association
Your cardiometabolic health is a measure of your risk for diabetes and heart disease, and is a good gauge of your overall health. Cardiometabolic health is determined by a set of conditions known as cardiometabolic factors. Manage cardiometabolic risk factors to prevent diabetes and heart disease.

Physical Inactivity Risk Factor
    Inactivity in those not disabled has an obvious visible effect, i.e., gaining weight. This was addressed in the section on overweight/obesity. What was not addressed is that the insulin receptor sites throughout the body may become suppressed due to the gain in weight. Insulin receptors are the receiving station of every cell for the circulating insulin needed for its intracellular function. There are multiple biologic regulators of the receptors and its post-receptor mechanisms in this complex chain of intracellular activity. It is an interesting concept that disruption of sufficient numbers of insulin receptor sites results in increased circulating insulin, hence hyperinsulinemia.

Exercise and diet were identified very early as the cornerstones of diabetes therapy, especially type 2 diabetes. Both exercise and diet have a direct effect on receptor reactivation, returning the circulating insulin to its normal level. Whenever additional support is needed, oral hypoglycemic medications can complete the transition to euinsulinemia.

High Blood Pressure/Essential Hypertension Risk Factor
Many years ago, the normal blood pressure (BP) was simply stated to be 100 mm Hg plus your age. If this were today's standard, one can only imagine the consequences if one were elderly. The current normal BP is less than 120/80 mm Hg. The terms *primary*, *idiopathic*, and/or *essential* mean without known cause. *Essential* has become the term most commonly used. Hypertension is the most common primary diagnosis in the United States; 35 million office visits have hypertension as the primary diagnosis.

The JNC 7 Report, 2003. *JAMA* 289, no. 19 (May 21): 2,560–72 provides a new guideline for hypertension prevention and management. The following are the key messages:
- In persons older than 50 years, systolic blood pressure of more than 140 mm Hg is a much more important cardiovascular disease (CVD) risk factor than diastolic BP.
- The risk of CVD, beginning at 65/75 mm Hg, doubles with each increment of 20/10 mm Hg; individuals who are normotensive at 55 years of age have a 90 percent lifetime risk for developing hypertension.
- Individuals with a systolic BP of 120 to 139 mm Hg or a diastolic BP of 80 to 89 mm Hg should be considered prehypertensive and require health-promoting lifestyle modifications to prevent CVD.
- Thiazide-type diuretics should be used in drug treatment for most patients with uncomplicated hypertension.
- Most patients with hypertension will require two or more antihypertensive medications.
- If BP is more than 20/10 mm Hg above goal BP, consideration should be given to initiating therapy with two agents, one of which usually should be a thiazide-type diuretic.
- The most effective therapy prescribed by the most careful clinician will control hypertension only if patients are motivated. Motivation improves when patients have positive experiences with and trust in the clinician.

The microangiopathy of the kidney is the anatomic pathology of hypertension. Hyperinsulinemia (insulin resistance) is the clinical pathology of hypertension. Hyperinsulinemia (insulin resistance) has been shown in population-based studies to predict the eventual development of essential hypertension. Conversely, patients with essential hypertension, as a group, are hyperinsulinemic (insulin resistant). "The Seventh Report of the Joint National Committee on Prevention, Detection, Evaluation, and Treatment of High Blood Pressure" fails to address the basic role of hyperinsulinemia (insulin resistance) and essential hypertension.   Essential hypertension, i.e. high blood pressure without known cause, is hyperinsulin, type 2 diabetes until proven otherwise by oral glucose tolerance with insulin assays. If YOU have high blood pressure or are being treated for high blood pressure, this means YOU. Medications need not be discontinued for the procedure. They may increase, but are not the cause of, your hyperinsulinemia. If you are to receive an oral glucose tolerance *without* the insulin assays, YOU are being short-changed as noted in every age group in Part 2.

High Blood Glucose Risk Factor
Normal = Fasting plasma glucose (FPG) less than 100 mg/d
Please see Chapter 2, Fasting Blood Sugar: What is Normal?

Smoking Risk Factor
The number of people still smoking in the United States and worldwide is staggering. Risk factors of smoking related to heart disease and diabetes are secondary to the well-established smoking-related pathology of emphysema and carcinoma of the lung. Over extended periods of time, emphysema of varying degrees is a 100 percent certainty, followed closely by a primary malignancy of the lung, the urinary bladder, and other malignancies.

If any of you now reading this book are smokers, please stop reading and give the book to a friend. If you are a smoker, you are not concerned about your future. This book, hopefully, is intended for those concerned about their future.

References:
1. Ferrannini, E., G. Buzzigoli, R. Bonadonna, et al. 1987. Insulin resistance in essential hypertension. *N Engl J Med* 317:350-57.
2. Chapter 2, Fasting Blood Glucose—What is Normal?
3. Chapter 14, Pathology of Type 2 Diabetes
4. Chapter 15, Clinical Pathology—Hyperinsulinemia

22

THE METABOLIC SYNDROME: WHAT IS IT?

THE WORLD HEALTH Organization (WHO) was the first organization to outline criteria for diagnosing the metabolic syndrome. It was proposed as a special designation to identify persons with the potential for diabetes. They were to have an impaired glucose tolerance, an impaired fasting glucose or insulin resistance identified by hyperinsulinemia euglycemic clamp procedure. According to the WHO, each component in their definition conveyed a greater cardiovascular disease risk (CVD), but when combined, the components became an even greater risk. The WHO's reason for diagnosing the metabolic syndrome was to identify persons at undue risk of CVD. The World Health Organization's definition of the Metabolic Syndrome states that the patient must have one of the following:

- Diabetes mellitus: fasting plasma glucose ≥126 mg/dl or 2-h postglucose load ≥200 mg/dl
- Impaired fasting glucose: fasting plasma glucose ≥110 mg/dl and ≤126 mg/dl and (if measured) 2-h postglucose load ≥140 mg/dl and less than 200 mg/dl
- Insulin resistance: glucose uptake below lowest quartile for background population under investigation under hyperinsulinemic euglycemic conditions
- Plus any two of the following:
  - Waist-to-hip ratio ≥0.9 in men, 0.85 in women, or BMI greater than 30
  - Triacylglycerols ≥150 mg/dl
  - HDL cholesterol ≤35 mg/dl in men and ≤39 mg/dl in women
  - Blood Pressure ≥140/90 mm Hg
  - Microalbuminuria

The Adult Treatment Panel III (ATPIII) provided its definition of the metabolic syndrome in 2001. The ATPIII was focused more on CVD risk and

less on type 2 diabetes. The Adult Treatment Panel III definition of the metabolic syndrome states that the patient must have any three of the following:
- Fasting glucose ≥110 mg/dl
- Waist circumference ≥40 inches in men and ≥35 inches in women
- Triacylglycerols ≥150 mg/dl
- HDL cholesterol ≤40 mg/dl in men and ≤50 mg/dl in women
- Blood Pressure ≥130/85 mg/dl

In 2005, the International Diabetes Federation (IDF) provided their definition of the Metabolic Syndrome. According to the IDF, for a diagnosis of Metabolic Syndrome, the patient must have:
- Central obesity, defined as waist circumference ≥94 cm for European men and ≥80 cm for European women, with ethnicity-specific values for other groups.

Plus any two of the following four factors:
- High triacylglycerol concentration: ≥150 mg/dl or specific treatment for this abnormality
- Low HDL cholesterol concentration: ≤40 mg/dl in males and ≤50 mg/dl in female or specific treatment for this lipid abnormality
- High blood pressure (BP): systolic ≥130 mm Hg or diastolic BP ≥85 mm Hg or treatment of previously diagnosed hypertension
- High fasting plasma glucose (FPG) concentration: ≥100 mg/dl or previously diagnosed type 2 diabetes. If FPG is above the stated values, an oral glucose tolerance is strongly recommended but is not necessary to define presence of the Syndrome.

A joint statement from the American Diabetes Association and the European Association for the Study of Diabetes (*Diabetes Care* 2005:28:2289–304) proposed the following guidelines:
- Providers should avoid labeling patients with the term *metabolic syndrome*
- Adults with any major CVD risk factor should be evaluated for the presence of other CVD risk factors
- All CVD risk factors should be individually and aggressively treated.

If your physician tells you that you have the *metabolic syndrome*, insist that he or she obtain and review the following reference: Reaven, G. J. 2006. The metabolic syndrome: Is this diagnosis necessary? *Am J Clin Nutr* 83:1237–47.

23

DIABETES AND IDIOPATHIC CARDIOMYOPATHY

THE PUBLICATION "DIABETES and Idiopathic Cardiomyopathy" is abstracted here for your perusal. (Bertoni, R. G., A.Tsai, E. K. Kasper, and F. L. Brancati. 2003. Diabetes and Idiopathic Cardiomyopathy: A Nationwide Case-Control Study. *Diabetes Care* 26, no. 10, October: 2791-95.) As a pathologist, I consider the article noteworthy, and my comments, therefore, are based on my pathology experiences. A more recent publication may also be of interest: Carmic, P. G., and F. Creas. 2007. Medical Progress: Coronary Microvascular Dysfunction. *N Engl J Med* (February 22):830–40.

Data source was from the Nationwide Inpatient Sample (NIS) collected under Healthcare Cost and Utilization Project 1988–1995. The NIS is designed to approximate a 20 percent sample of nonfederal short-term general and specialty hospitals in the U. S. There were 90,000+ cases coded as primary cardiomyopathy. Half were coded as ischemic heart disease and the other half as idiopathic cardiomyopathy (ICM). Conclusions:

1. Hospitalizations occurred at a higher rate among individuals with diabetes.
2. Diabetes was associated with ICM, independent of age, gender, income, or hypertension.
3. The association was strongest among discharges with microvascular complications of diabetes.
4. Diabetes is significantly associated with nonischemic systolic dysfunction.
5. Diabetes-related ICM occurs more frequently than had been suspected.

In "Diabetes Mellitus and Congestive Heart Failure," the authors cite a reference that hyperinsulinemia (insulin resistance) is associated with diabetes and impaired endothelial function leading to heart muscle dysfunction as a consequence of compromised myocardial blood flow (Solang, L., K. Malmberg, and L. Ryden. 1999. *Eur Heart J* 20: 789-95). It is a known fact that myocardial ischemia does occur. It is not always due to the major arteries of the heart, but also to the capillaries. The capillaries, which are lined by endothelium located throughout the myocardium, are the target of hyperinsulinemia; hence, type 2 diabetes pathology. The February 2007 issue of *National Geographic* features an article entitled, "Healing the Heart." The photos illustrating the large and medium-sized arteries are excellent.

In the field of pathology, capillary blood flow of the heart has been known for some time. The Armed Forces Institute of Pathology has illustrated, by specific techniques, the tiniest branching capillaries deep within and throughout the myocardium. They appear like the end segments of the delicate roots of a plant. In my experience as a pathologist, microscopic examination of the heart in clinical heart failure with or without cardiomyopathy and in the absence of significant coronary arteriosclerotic narrowing of the lumen, have revealed focal, thread-like markings within the muscle fibers. For want of a better term, I had considered this indicative of capillary ischemia. The two articles cited above address clinical cardiomyopathy with descriptive terms of idiopathic cardiomyopathy and coronary microvascular dysfunction. Both studies are devoid of autopsy pathology of the heart for possible correlation with their clinical concepts.

Since the 1970s, the aftermath of this drought of postmortem examinations throughout the U. S. has resulted in a relative halt to expansion of knowledge of the pathology of the heart. MRI and other similar examination techniques are not equivalent to autopsy examination. This autopsy drought in the U. S. is of major clinical consequence in the pathology of the heart in diabetes.

24

HYPERINSULINEMIA VS. INSULIN RESISTANCE

Insulin resistance is a concept—a concept of increased insulin production.
Hyperinsulinemia is increased insulin—determined by direct measurement.
Insulin resistance is *hyperinsulinemia*.

In Chapter 7, the Yalow-Berson Contribution, the introduction of the term *insulin resistance* is described. A brief review is essentially this: Soon after insulin therapy was available, it was noted that antibodies to the insulin, which was a foreign protein to the body coming from animals, occurred. In some instances, this required a marked increasing of the patient's insulin dose. This phenomenon was called *insulin resistance*. After the introduction of the radioimmunoassay by Yalow and Berson, the increased insulin (*hyperinsulinemia*) identified in type 2 diabetes, for want of a better term, was also referred to as *insulin resistance*.

With limited experience with the oral glucose tolerance and insulin assays, clinical investigations contrived various research procedures to "measure" insulin resistance. These procedures consisted mainly of the insulin suppression test to measure resistance to insulin-mediated glucose uptake, the euglycemic hyperinsulinemia clamp technique, and the hyperglycemic clamp technique. The results were interpreted as degrees of insulin resistance. The procedures were not technically applicable for clinical utilization nor did they identify a relationship to hyperinsulinemia.

A mathematical model of the glucose:insulin interactions has been used to indicate the degree to which they combine to give hyperglycemia with low, normal, or raised basal plasma insulin concentrations. (D. R. Matthews, J. P. Treacher, A. S. Rudenski, B. A. Naylor, J. R. Hosker and R. C. Turner. 1985. Homeostasis Model Assessment: insulin resistance and beta-cell function from fasting plasma glucose and insulin concentration in man. Diabetes Research Laboratories, Radcliffe Infirmary, Oxford, UK. *Diabetologia* 28:412–19.) The Homeostasis Model Assessment of insulin resistance (HOMA-IR) formula:

$$\text{HOMA-IR} = \text{fasting insulin } (\mu U/ml) \times \frac{\underline{\text{fasting plasma glucose}} \text{ (mmol/l)}}{22.5}$$

Plasma glucose in mg/dl is converted to mmol/l by mg/dl x 0.05551 = mmol/l. A key word in the formula is assessment. The numbers produced are relative and are *not* quantitative measurements. This mathematical hypothesis was tested on a limited number of persons—mainly 12 normal (23–67 years) and 11 type 2 diabetes (46–68 years) by euglycemic clamp, hyperglycemic clamp, and I.V. glucose tolerance. Oral glucose tolerances with insulin assays for a direct measurement of insulin were not performed.

The assessment or determination of insulin resistance (hyperinsulinemia) by innovative research methodologies and/or mathematical projection by fasting insulin and fasting glucoses are deficient in the identification of hyperinsulinemia. There is a sharp contrast to the direct measurement of insulin with the oral glucose tolerance not limited to a few hundred examinations but in 14,384 examinations as so noted in Table 4 (See Chapter 13).

Hyperinsulinemia Is Insulin Resistance.

They Are Not Combatants.

They Are One And The Same.

Part Two

Age Distribution of 14,384 Oral Glucose Tolerances With Insulin Assays

3–13 through 81–90+ year age group

25

3–13 Age Group

N = 117
Normal Glucose Tolerance
N = 104
Impaired Glucose Tolerance
N = 7
Diabetes Mellitus Glucose Tolerance
N = 6

Before reviewing the oral glucose tolerance 75-g load or equivalent with insulin assays on the 117 in the 3–13 year old age group and the 651 in the 14–20 year old age group, I have abstracted pertinent references for your perusal.

(Fajans, S. S., G. I. Bell, and K. S. Polonsky. 2001. Molecular mechanisms and clinical pathophysiology of maturity-onset diabetes of the young. *N Engl J Med* 345, no. 1, September 27.) The article is a review of basic research plus the authors' clinical views and projections. Maturity-Onset Diabetes of the Young (MODY) is a mild asymptomatic hyperglycemia in non-obese children, adolescents, and young adults who have a prominent family history of diabetes, often in successive generations. The pattern is consistent with an autosomal dominant mode of inheritance. MODY can result from mutations of any one of at least six different genes labeled MODY 1–6. To date, more than 120 mutations in this gene have been identified. Genetic screening for MODY is only applicable in a research setting. Commercial tests are not available. Hyperinsulinemia (insulin resistance) is not addressed in their review. The possible clinical impact of MODY identification has not been confirmed, whereas the merit of hyperinsulinemia, type 2 diabetes has been established.

Dr. Francine R. Kaufman is head of the Division of Endocrinology, Diabetes and Metabolism at Children's Hospital, Los Angeles, and a professor of pediatrics at the Keck School of Medicine of the University of California. She is a past president of the American Diabetes Association. Her book, *Diabesity. The Obesity-Diabetes Epidemic that Threatens American—And What We Must Do to Stop It*. New York: Bantam Books, 2005 is a must read, especially for all those under 20 years of age. It is divided into three parts: Part 1—The Devil is Diabetes; Part 2—The Evolution of our Destruction; and Part 3—Engines of Change. *Diabesity* is an easy read. Once you start, you will not want to put it down. In 2002, Dr. Kaufman alerted the membership of the American Diabetes Association that type 2 diabetes was being described as a "new epidemic" in the American Pediatric population. (Kaufman, F. R. 2002. Type 2 diabetes in children and young adults!—A "New Epidemic." *Clin Diabetes* 20:217-18.)

Another reference: Kraft, J. R. "Glucose/insulin tolerance testing for the prospective management of diabetes/atherosclerosis with prime focus on childhood." In: U. P. Merten and J. Linder, eds. *Pathology—A Medical Specialty. Proceedings of the 10th Triennial World Congress of Anatomic and Clinical Patholog.* 1978. Rio de Janeiro, Brazil (September 25–29, 1978). World Association of Societies of Pathology, Cologne, W Germany, 1979, pp. 608-11. "Approaching the problem of atherosclerosis (heart disease, hypertension, etc.) at age 60 has far less potential of prevention than at age 10–15. Prospective management applicable to atherosclerosis prevention of all known etiological factors utilizing effective diabetes identification and diet therapy must be directed towards childhood and young adults when potential benefit of therapeutic intervention is greatest."

A more recent reference is the following: Presence of Diabetes Risk Factors in a Large U. S. Eighth-Grade Cohort. The STOPP-T2o Study Group. *Diabetes Care* 29, no. 2 (February 2006). The objective of this study of 1,740 eighth-grade students conducted in 12 middle schools was to determine the prevalence of diabetes, prediabetes, and diabetes risk factors. The students were predominantly minority. The conclusions of this study group were the identification of a high prevalence of risk factors for diabetes. This included impaired fasting glucose (greater than 100 mg/dl), hyperinsulinemia suggestive of insulin resistance, fasting insulins greater than 30 microunits/ml, and overweight. They further concluded that middle schools are appropriate targets for population-based efforts to decrease overweight and diabetes risk. This study emphasized that hyperinsulinemia (insulin resistance) is a major risk factor for type 2 diabetes in the young.

3–13 Age Group/N = 117

- The mean age was 10 years. One child less than 6 years of age was 3 years old who tested normal, nondiabetic.
- There were 70 girls and 47 boys.
- The weights of the children were given for the purpose of determining the 75-g glucose load equivalent.
- The glucose tolerances with insulin assays were ordered by their physicians to exclude or identify prediabetes or diabetes.
- The examinations were critiqued by the American Diabetes Association guidelines for fasting blood glucose (FBG) and oral glucose tolerance (OGT).

NGT = 104
    51 = normal insulin, nondiabetes   (49%)
    53 = hyperinsulin type 2 diabetes   (51%)

IGT = 7
    4 = normal insulin, nondiabetes   (57%)
    3 = hyperinsulin type 2 diabetes   (43%)

DMGT = 6
    4 = hypoinsulin type 1 diabetes (potential)   (67%)
    2 = hyperinsulin type 2 diabetes   (33%)

Normal, nondiabetes = 47%   (55 of 117)
Hyperinsulinemia, type 2 diabetes = 50%   (58 of 117)
Hypoinsulinemia, type 1 diabetes (potential) = 3%   (4 of 117)

Fasting Blood Glucose less than 100 mg/dl:
    NGT = 97   or 93% of   104
    IGT = 4   or 60% of   7
    DMGT = 0   or 0% of   <u>6</u>
                                          117

The 2006 and 2007 American Diabetes Association guidelines stated that only FBG greater than 100 mg/dl should be further tested by oral glucose tolerance. Therefore:

- Only 16 with FBG greater than 100 mg/dl would have been tested by oral glucose tolerance.
- 101 of the 117 in this 3–13 year old age group would not have been tested, leaving their prediabetes or diabetes or nondiabetes status unknown.
- The oral glucose tolerance (OGT) without insulin assay for the identification of increased insulin (hyperinsulin) or low insulin (hypoinsulin) or normal insulin (euinsulin) is incomplete.
- With the oral glucose tolerance and insulin assays, none of the 3–13 year age group were excluded from diabetes evaluation.

26

14–20 Age Group

N = 651
Normal Glucose Tolerance
N = 569
Impaired Glucose Tolerance
N = 65
Diabetes Mellitus Glucose Tolerance
N = 17

- The mean age was 16 years.
- There were 495 girls and 156 boys.
- BMI for overweight was not determined.
- All received the 75-g glucose load for the oral glucose/insulin tolerance test.
- Referring physicians ordered the oral glucose tolerance with insulin assays to identify or exclude prediabetes or diabetes.
- The results of the examinations were critiqued with the American Diabetes Association guidelines for fasting blood sugar and oral glucose tolerance (2007).

NGT = 569
        126 = normal insulin nondiabetes   (22%)
        443 = hyperinsulin type 2 diabetes   (78%)

IGT = 65
        3 = normal insulin (5%)
        62 = hyperinsulin type 2 diabetes   (95%)

DMGT = 17
    4 = hypoinsulin type 1 diabetes (potential)   (24%)
    13 = hyperinsulin type 2 diabetes   (76%)

Hyperinsulinemia, type 2 diabetes = 79.5%
Normal insulin, nondiabetes = 19.8%
Hypoinsulin, type 1 diabetes (potential) = 0.6%

Fasting Blood Glucose less than 100 mg/dl:
    NGT = 529   or 93% of 569
    IGT = 16   or 24% of 65
    DMGT = 3   or 19% of <u>17</u>
                                 651

The ADA guidelines limit further testing by oral glucose tolerance to those with FBG greater than 100 mg/dl. This limits it to only 103 of the 651 in this 14–20 year age group. Therefore, 548 or 84 percent of this group would not be tested, leaving their prediabetes or diabetes or nondiabetes status unknown. The oral glucose tolerance without insulin assay in all age groups for the identification of increased insulin (hyperinsulin) or low insulin (hypoinsulin) or normal insulin (euinsulin) is incomplete. With the oral glucose tolerance including the insulin assays, none of the 651 in this 14–20 year old age group were excluded from prediabetes or diabetes evaluation.

27

21–30 Age Group

N = 3720
Normal Glucose Tolerance
N = 3106
Impaired Glucose Tolerance
N = 485
Diabetes Mellitus Glucose Tolerance
N = 129

- The mean age was 25.5 years.
- There were 3,188 women and 532 men.
- All received the 100-g glucose load for the oral glucose tolerance.
- Staff physicians ordered the glucose tolerance with insulin assays to determine nondiabetes, prediabetes, diabetes, or Gestational Diabetes.
- The results of the examinations were critiqued with the American Diabetes Association guidelines for fasting blood glucose and oral glucose tolerance.
- Gestational Diabetes is reviewed in Chapter 17.

NGT = 3106
        694 = normal insulin nondiabetes   (22%)
        2412 = hyperinsulin type 2 diabetes   (78%)
IGT = 485
        24 = normal insulin   (5%)
        461 = hyperinsulin type 2 diabetes   (95%)
DMGT = 129
        20 = hypoinsulin type 1 diabetes, potential   (16%)
        109 = hyperinsulin type 2 diabetes   (84%)

Hyperinsulinemia type 2 diabetes = 80% of 3,720
Type 1 diabetes (potential) = 0.2%
Normal insulin, nondiabetes = 19.8%

Fasting Blood Glucose less than 100 mg/dl:
    NGT = 93%   or 2889 of 3106
    IGT = 60%   or 291 of 485
    DMGT = 20%   <u>or 26 of 129</u>
                           3206 of 3720

The ADA fasting blood criteria eliminates 86 percent of the 3,720 in the 21–30 age group from further testing by oral glucose tolerance. Only those with FBG greater than 100 mg/dl would be tested. This would consist of:

    217 of the   3106 NGT
    194 of the   485 IGT
    <u>103 of the</u>   <u>129 DMGT</u>
    514 of   3720

The limitations of the oral glucose tolerance without insulin assays cannot be overemphasized. Without the insulin assay, the dynamic insulin status of normal, increased (hyperinsulin), or low (hypoinsulin) cannot be determined. The importance to the patient of hyperinsulinemia, type 2 diabetes identification in its earliest stages of prediabetes cannot be overemphasized. Please review Chapter 14 on the pathology of type 2 diabetes.

28

31–40 AGE GROUP

N = 2695
Normal Glucose Tolerance
NGT = 2049
Impaired Glucose Tolerance
IGT = 456
Diabetes Mellitus Glucose Tolerance
DMGT = 190

- The mean age was 35.6 years.
- There were 2,281 women and 414 men.
- All received the 100-g glucose load for the oral glucose tolerance with insulin assays.
- Referring physicians ordered the examination to exclude or identify prediabetes or diabetes.
- The results of the examination were critiqued with the American Diabetes Association guidelines updated for 2006 and 2007 for fasting blood glucose and the oral glucose tolerance.

NGT = 2049
    471 = normal insulin nondiabetes
    1578 = hyperinsulin, type 2 diabetes

IGT = 456
    23 = normal insulin
    433 = hyperinsulin, type 2 diabetes

DMGT = 190
    6 = hypoinsulin (low insulin) type 1 diabetes, potential
    184 = hyperinsulin, type 2 diabetes.

Hyperinsulinemia is type 2 diabetes not only identified in the DMGT, but also in the IGT and the NGT. In this 31–40 age group, 81 percent were type 2 diabetes, hyperinsulinemia, 18 percent were nondiabetic, and 0.2 percent were type 1 diabetes, potential.

Fasting Blood Sugar less than 100 mg/dl (FBG):
NGT =   1906   or 93% of 2049   = normal FBG
IGT =   274   or 60% of 456   = normal FBG
DMGT =   38   or 20% of 190   = normal FBG
         2218   2695

ADA guidelines: FBG less than 100 mg/dl (normal) need not be tested further by oral glucose tolerance. This guideline would separate 82 percent or 2, 218 of the 2,695 persons in this 31–40 age group from further testing by oral glucose tolerance. Again, the American Diabetes Association guidelines for FBG and oral glucose tolerance without insulin assays fail to identify hyperinsulinemia, type 2 diabetes, not only in the DMGT but also in the IGT and the NGT.

If this is your age group, and you are tested by an oral glucose tolerance with insulin assays, you will be in one of these categories—NGT, IGT, or DMGT. What is your choice?

29

41–50 AGE GROUP

N = 1924
Normal Glucose Tolerance
NGT = 1231
Impaired Glucose Tolerance
IGT = 373
Diabetes Mellitus Glucose Tolerance
DMGT = 320

- The mean age was 45.8 years.
- There were 1,193 women and 731 men.
- All receive the 100-g glucose load for the oral glucose tolerance with insulin assays.
- The examinations were ordered by their physicians to identify or exclude prediabetes or diabetes.
- The results were critiqued with the American Diabetes Association guidelines (2006 and 2007) for fasting blood sugar and oral glucose tolerance.

NGT = 1231
    309 = normal insulin nondiabetes
    922 = hyperinsulin type 2 diabetes
IGT = 373
    19 = normal insulin nondiabetes
    354 = hyperinsulin type 2 diabetes
DMGT = 320
    24 = hypoinsulin, type 1 diabetes, potential
    296 = hyperinsulin, type 2 diabetes

Hyperinsulinemia is type 2 diabetes.

Hypoinsulinemia (low response) is type 1 diabetes, potential, with DMGT.

Normal insulin (euinsulinemia) is nondiabetes with NGT and IGT.

Fasting Blood Sugar less than 100 mg/dl (FBG):

```
        NGT =    1145    or 93% of  1231   = normal FBG
        IGT =     224    or 60% of   373   = normal FBG
        DMGT =    64     or 20% of   320   = normal FBG
                 1433               1924
```

There are 1,433 or 74 percent of the 1,924 persons in this 41–50 age group with "normal" fasting blood sugars. According to ADA guidelines, they would not need an oral glucose tolerance. Hyperinsulinemia is type 2 diabetes by oral glucose tolerance with insulin assays in the DMGT, the IGT, and the NGT. The oral glucose tolerance without insulin assay is incomplete.

```
        NGT = 922      or 75% of 1231 = type 2 diabetes
        IGT = 354      or 95% of 373 = type 2 diabetes
        DMGT = 296     or 93% of 320 = type 2 diabetes
```

This age group of 41–50 years is when the pathology of prediabetes and diabetes may begin to blossom. Please review Chapter 14, Pathology of Type 2 Diabetes. Is it too late to be concerned about your future? Absolutely not! Review the chapter on risk factors and let the concern for your future begin today.

30

51–60 AGE GROUP

N = 2413
Normal Glucose Tolerance
N = 1302
Impaired Glucose Tolerance
N = 603
Diabetes Mellitus Glucose Tolerance
N = 508

- The mean age was 56.0 years.
- There were 1,924 women and 489 men.
- The 100-g glucose load for oral glucose tolerance with insulin assay was received by all.
- The procedure was ordered by their physicians to exclude or diagnose prediabetes or diabetes.
- The results were critiqued with the American Diabetes Association guidelines for fasting blood glucose and oral glucose tolerance.

NGT = 1302
        252 = normal insulin nondiabetes
        1050 = hyperinsulin type 2 diabetes
IGT = 603
        30 = normal insulin nondiabetes
        573 = hyperinsulin type 2 diabetes
DMGT = 508
        46 = hypoinsulin (low insulin) type 1 diabetes, potential
        462 = hyperinsulin, type 2 diabetes

In every age group, hyperinsulinemia is type 2 diabetes.

```
NGT  =   1050    or 81% of  1302  = type 2 diabetes
IGT  =    573    or 95% of   603  = type 2 diabetes
DMGT = _462_     or 91% of  _508_ = type 2 diabetes
         2085               2413
```

2,085 or 86% = type 2 diabetes.

Fasting blood Glucose less than 100 mg/dl (FBG):
```
NGT  =   1211    or 93% of  1302  = normal FBG
IGT  =    362    or 60% of   603  = normal FBG
DMGT = _102_     or 20% of  _508_ = normal FBG
         1675               2413
```

ADA Guidelines: FBG less than 100 mg/dl (normal) need not be further tested by oral glucose tolerance. If this had been applied to this study, 69 percent or 1,675 of the 2,413 in this age group of 51–60 would not have been tested by oral glucose tolerance, let alone oral glucose tolerance with insulin assay. The limitations of the ADA guidelines are again highlighted as incomplete.

31

61–70 Age Group

N = 1720
Normal Glucose Tolerance
N = 827
Impaired Glucose Tolerance
N = 464
Diabetes Mellitus Glucose Tolerance
N = 429

- The mean age was 64 years.
- There were 925 women and 795 men.
- The 100-g glucose load for the oral glucose tolerance with insulin assay was received by all.
- The examinations were ordered by their physicians to identify or exclude prediabetes and/or diabetes.
- The results were critiqued with the American Diabetes Association guidelines (2006–2007) for fasting blood sugar and the oral glucose tolerance.

NGT = 827
       135 = normal insulin, nondiabetes
       692 = hyperinsulin, type 2 diabetes
IGT = 464
       23 = normal insulin, nondiabetes
       441 = hyperinsulin, type 2 diabetes
DMGT = 429
       39 = hypoinsulin, type 1 diabetes, potential
       390 = hyperinsulin, type 2 diabetes

Hyperinsulinemia is type 2 diabetes.

```
NGT  =   692    or 84% of  827   = type 2 diabetes
IGT  =   441    or 95% of  464   = type 2 diabetes
DMGT =   390    or 91% of  429   = type 2 diabetes
         1523              1720
```

Fasting Blood Sugar less than 100 mg/dl (FBG):
```
NGT  =   769    or 93% of  827   = normal FBG
IGT  =   278    or 60% of  464   = normal FBG
DMGT =    86    or 20% of  429   = normal FBG
         1133             1720
```

The ADA guidelines for FBG remain unchanged (2007). FBG less than 100 mg/dl (normal) need not be further tested unless there are clinical findings of diabetes. Applying this guideline, 66 percent of the 61–70 age group would not have been tested by oral glucose tolerance with insulin assays. The limitations of the ADA guidelines (2007) for FBG and oral glucose tolerance without insulin assays are again demonstrated.

The following current reference is given, which is of concern to all of us elderly: Seloin, E., J. Curesh, and F. Brancati. 2006. "The burden and treatment of diabetes in elderly individuals in the U. S." *Diabetes Care* 29, no. 11 (November): 2414–19. The number of people age 65 or older is increasing markedly. They represented 12 percent of the U. S. population in the year 2000, and this proportion is expected to grow to almost 20 percent by the year 2020 (up to 55 million people). Diabetes and its related problems of obesity, hyperinsulinemia, and impaired glucose tolerance (which is prediabetes) are growing health care problems in the U. S. The cumulative lifetime incidence of diabetes is estimated to increase by 30 percent. *Age is a known risk factor for diabetes.*

32

71–80 AGE GROUP

N = 932
Normal Glucose Tolerance
N = 345
Impaired Glucose Tolerance
N = 261
Diabetes Mellitus Glucose Tolerance
N = 326

- The mean age was 76 years.
- There were 634 women and 298 men.
- The 100-g glucose load for the oral glucose tolerance with insulin assays was received by all.
- Their physicians ordered this examination to exclude or identify prediabetes or diabetes.
- The results of the examinations for the 932 senior citizens in this 71–80 age group were critiqued with the American Diabetes Association guidelines for fasting blood glucose (FBG) and oral glucose tolerance (2007).

NGT = 345
        64 normal insulin, nondiabetes
        281 hyperinsulin, type 2 diabetes
IGT = 261
        13 normal insulin, nondiabetes
        248 hyperinsulin, type 2 diabetes
DMGT = 326
        35 hypoinsulin (low insulin), type 1 diabetes, potential
        291 hyperinsulin, type 2 diabetes

Hyperinsulinemia is type 2 diabetes, not only with DMGT, but also with the IGT and the NGT—88 percent or 820 of the 932 persons were type 2 diabetes.

Fasting Blood Sugar less than 100 mg/dl (FBG):

NGT =	321	or 93% of	345	= normal FBG
IGT =	156	or 60% of	261	= normal FBG
DMGT =	65	or 20% of	326	= normal FBG
	542		932	

The ADA guidelines (2007): FBG "normal," less than 100 mg/dl, separated 542 of the 932 (58%) in this 71–80 age group that would not be further evaluated by oral glucose tolerance unless there were clinical indications of diabetes. Irrespective of age, the ADA guidelines for normal fasting blood sugar and oral glucose tolerance without insulin assays, which are essential for hyperinsulinemia identification, are incomplete.

Many of the elderly may consider themselves to be home free from becoming diabetic. *Not so!* The ADA standard for the diabetes mellitus glucose tolerance which requires a second hour glucose level of greater than 200 mg/dl (75-g glucose load) is designated diabetes (DMGT). In this age group, you will note that *326 of the 932 (35%) seniors were identified DMGT.* Without the insulin assays, type 1 diabetes and type 2 diabetes cannot be determined. However, the insulin assays with the oral glucose tolerance identified *35 of the 326 with DMGT to be insulin deficient (11%), type 1 diabetes, potential.* In addition, 291 of the 326 DMGT (89%) were type 2 diabetes.

How can this be? *The clinical silence of high blood sugars is an enigma of diabetes.* This silence accounts for the multiple millions of people worldwide with diabetes who don't know they have it. If you are in this age group and have so far been free of much of the pathology of type 2 diabetes, continue to contain your risks. The choice is yours.

33

81–90+ Age Group

N = 212
Normal Glucose Tolerance
N = 65
Impaired Glucose Tolerance
N = 61
Diabetes Mellitus Glucose Tolerance
N = 86

- The mean age was 84 years.
- There were 184 women and 28 men.
- Each received the 100-g glucose load for the oral glucose tolerance with insulin assays.
- Their physicians ordered the examinations to exclude diabetes for whatever reason known only by the patient and the physician.
- The results in the examinations performed on the 212 senior citizens in this grand age of 81–90+ were critiqued with the American Diabetes Association guidelines (2007) for fasting blood sugar (FBG) and oral glucose tolerance.

NGT = 65
        10 = normal insulin, nondiabetes
        55 = hyperinsulin, type 2 diabetes
IGT = 61
        3 = normal insulin, nondiabetes
        58 = hyperinsulin, type 2 diabetes
DMGT = 86
        8 = hypoinsulin (low insulin), type 1 diabetes, potential
        78 = hyperinsulin, type 2 diabetes

Hyperinsulinemia is type 2 diabetes, not only in the DMGT, but also in the IGT and the NGT.

> 191 or 90% of the 212 = type 2 diabetes
> 13 or 6% of the 212 = nondiabetes
> 8 or 4% of the 212 = type 1 diabetes, potential

Fasting Blood Sugar less than 100 ml/dl (FBG):
> NGT = 59 or 90% of 65 = normal FBG
> IGT = 36 or 59% of 61 = normal FBG
> DMGT = 17 or 20% of 86 = normal FBG
> 112 212

ADA guidelines (2007): FBG "normal," less than 100 mg/dl, separated 112 of the 212 in this super senior citizen age group of 80–90+ that would not need further testing by oral glucose tolerance. The exception would be if any indicators of diabetes were evident. This guideline would result in 53 percent of the 212 in the 80–90+ age group not being evaluated by an oral glucose tolerance with insulin assay. The ADA guidelines for fasting blood sugar and oral glucose tolerances without the insulin assay are incomplete in every age group, including the 80–90+ group, which has been blessed with longevity.

The diagnosis of diabetes may come as a surprise to persons in this age 80–90+ group. This was true for my Grandmother K., who was first diagnosed as a diabetic at 82 years of age. The insulin therapy was helpful; nevertheless, she expired due to congestive heart failure two years later. The 40 percent of the 212 with DMGT may also have been surprised. This could be particularly true for the eight with insulin deficiency, type 1 diabetes, potential, thereby making them candidates for insulin therapy. Although I am not one of the 212, I have empathy for them, because as of today, I am right in the middle of this age group.

34

DIABETES: A WORLDWIDE PLAGUE FACING THE CHALLENGE

ACCORDING TO THE International Diabetes Federation (the counterpart of the American Diabetes Association), the number of people around the world suffering from diabetes has skyrocketed in the past two decades, from 30 million to 230 million. China now has the largest number of diabetics over age 20, and India is second. In the Middle East, the Federation estimates the diabetic population to be between 12 and 20 percent. These estimates are only the tip of the iceberg. The "silent" diabetics with "normal" fasting blood sugars, if tested by an oral glucose tolerance, will have 2-h sugars, in the diabetes range. This will multiply their numbers of diabetics just as it has in the U. S. The International Diabetes Federation (IDF) is seeking a U. N. resolution to recognize the seriousness of the worldwide problem.

Challenge #1

The IDF and the ADA do not as yet fully agree on the incidence of prediabetes and diabetes occurring with "normal" fasting blood sugar. There is a common ground, however, with impaired fasting sugar (IFG). This is encouraging. Whether in Europe or the United States, it is essential that insulin assays be part of the oral glucose tolerance in the testing of those with impaired fasting sugar, i.e., greater than 100 mg/dl. Without the insulin assays, an impact on the Diabetes Plague will not begin.

The 14,384 examinations, which are unequaled, have repeatedly affirmed in every age group that the oral glucose tolerance without insulin assays for the identification of increased insulin (hyperinsulin) or low insulin (hypoinsulin) or normal insulin (euinsulin) in relation to prediabetes and diabetes is incomplete.

Challenge #2

In recent times, the clinical application of the oral glucose tolerance with insulin assay has been minimal. Many pathologists and most clinicians, including professors from distinguished universities, have little to zero personal experience with it. In order for their opinions to have credibility regarding the procedure and its interpretation, a randomized personal experience of a minimum of one thousand examinations would suffice. Once this experience has been achieved, the reproducibility of the oral glucose tolerance with insulin assay will be self- evident.

Challenge #3

How early should diabetes be treated? This may appear to be a ridiculous question, and that it is. It has been a basic principle of medicine since Hippocrates' time that the earliest diagnosis provides the opportunity for treatment with the greatest chance for cure.

In tumor pathology, when the microscopic identification of the tumor revealed that it was still confined, it was designated in-situ, i.e., in place. This term was first introduced into pathology terminology in biopsies of the cervix when the carcinoma was limited to the epithelium—hence, carcinoma in-situ. In most instances, this had been preceded by Pap smears showing atypical exfoliated cells prior to the biopsy confirmation.

In 1974 and 1975, our oral glucose tolerances with insulin assays demonstrated that hyperinsulinemia is type 2 diabetes. This was not only of major importance with the diabetes mellitus glucose tolerances but also with the impaired glucose tolerances and especially with the normal glucose tolerances. Even though these initial findings were limited to only 3,650 examinations, they were convincing to my clinical colleagues and to me. The findings have been concurred over and over again in the subsequent 14,384 examinations. As a pathologist, I considered it quite apropos and logical to designate the hyperinsulinemia, type 2 diabetes with the normal glucose tolerance, "diabetes mellitus in-situ (occult diabetes)." *Laboratory Medicine* 6, no. 2 (February 1975).

Challenge #4

In the October 13, 2006 *Wall Street Journal*, p. B1, "Firms Study Drugs to Help Avert Diabetes" was featured. It was stated that a growing number of drug makers and doctors are examining whether medications can help prevent the disease in others who are at risk of developing it, thus potentially creating a vast new market for the pharmaceutical industry.

The FDA and others raise the question—why use a prescription drug to avert a disease that studies show can often be effectively "prevented" through a careful diet and exercise? The ADA recommends weight loss and exercise, and that drug therapy should not be routinely used to prevent diabetes until there is more information about its cost-effectiveness. After all, how much is a life worth—especially yours? The supporters of early treatment state that it is not a case of either/or. It is both. You, the reader, must remember that the diabetes organizations and the drug industry, when using the term "diabetes," are addressing the hyperglycemic (late phase), type 2 diabetes. It is their mutual goal to prevent this phase, hoping to delay or eliminate the clinical pathology of diabetes. This is a good time to review Chapter 14, Pathology of Type 2 Diabetes. It is quite evident that representatives of the diabetes organizations and the drug makers are not pathologists.

Without question, nutritional management, weight control, and exercise are the cornerstones for diabetes therapy. In due time, drug therapy will have a place in the treatment of diabetes mellitus in-situ (occult diabetes). The time has come for the supporters of early treatment to apply their support to the earliest diagnosis which is hyperinsulinemia, type 2 diabetes with normal glucose tolerance. *The impact on the Diabetes Plague will be staggering.*

Challenge #5

Is the ADA facing the challenge of the diabetes epidemic? Indeed they are! The ADA has launched a dramatic ad campaign to draw attention to the needed fight against diabetes. Several ads highlight the following:
- 82,000 Americans lost a leg because of diabetes last year.
- Every 21 seconds, another American is diagnosed with diabetes.
- 224,092 American die from diabetes-related illnesses each year.

The ads emphasize that time is of the essence. They urge Congress to increase funding for diabetes management and research. *Diabetes Care*, March 2007, features a consensus report reaffirming the ADA position, essentially unchanged—on IFG (impaired fasting glucose, i.e., values greater than 100 mg/dl and less than 126 mg/dl) and IGT (impaired glucose tolerance, i.e., second hour after a 75-g glucose load greater than 140 mg/dl and less than 200 mg/dl). You may obtain a copy of this report at the following website: www.care.diabetesjournals.org.

Neither the dramatic ads nor the recent ADA guidelines (March 2007) on IFG and IGT address the earliest identification of type 2 diabetes, hyperinsulinemia by normal glucose tolerance with insulin assays. A question you must ask: Will the ADA, through its membership, ever recognize and emphasize the importance of the earliest identification of diabetes? The answer is YES, of course they will! In due time, YOU, the PUBLIC, will demand it.

Challenge #6

Will you ever, as a type 2 diabetic, need to receive insulin? Of course you will!! There is important news for you! The American Diabetes Association now recommends adding insulin earlier in your treatment program. If your blood sugars are not under control after two to three months of diet, exercise, and oral medications, absolutely YOU need the addition of insulin. Why, you must ask, is it necessary to wait up to three months, observing the blood sugars out of control, before adding insulin? It is not necessary! An oral glucose tolerance with insulin assays will determine your insulin needs now!

In Table 4, Chapter 13, up to 24 percent of the DMGT with fasting blood sugars greater than 130 mg/dl had low insulins, identifying the need of insulin in their diabetes management. By adding insulin earlier as part of your diabetes program, as the American Diabetes Association recommends, lowering of your blood sugar levels will occur. Hopefully, this will delay the ongoing pathology of your type 2 diabetes. (See Chapter 14.)

Challenge #7

Are 2-h oral glucose tolerances with insulin assays equal to the standard 3-h examination? Yes, they can be!
1) Interpretation based upon American Diabetes Association guidelines for the oral glucose tolerance and insulin assay identification of normal (euinsulin), increased (hyperinsulin), and low (hypoinsulin)—based upon the 14,000+ examinations—provide not only screening but also diagnostic clinical data.
2) A two-hour procedure based upon oral glucose tolerance with insulin assays was proposed in 1990. (Kraft, J. R. and K. T. Sie. 1990. Hyperinsulin/insulin resistant NIDDM state identification; a practical screening procedure. *Diabetes* 39 Suppl: 695.) The 2-h examination was to be like the 3-h oral glucose tolerance with insulin assays, except no 3-h specimen was obtained. Just as fasting and second-hour

glucoses are a key to their classification, the fasting and second-hour insulin assays are equally essential for the classification and completion of the oral glucose tolerance examination.

3) In Chapter 11, Normal Fasting Insulin: What is Normal?, Table 2 identifies the distribution in the 14,000+ oral glucose tolerances with insulin assays. Fasting insulins greater than 30 microunits per milliliter diagnostic of hyperinsulinemia ranged from 5% in the NGT and IGT to 16% in the DMGT. The overall percentage in the 14,000+ examinations is 8%. Within the above incidence, fasting insulin can identify hyperinsulinemia, type 2 diabetes.

4) The second-hour insulin is key to the modified 2-h examination for values greater than 60 microunits per milliliter are diagnostic of hyperinsulinemia. In Table 3 of Chapter 12, Dynamic Insulin Patterns, *70% of the 14000+ examinations were greater than 60 microunits*. Within this incidence, credence is given to the 2-h examination. With normal fasting insulins in the 14,000+ examinations, the second-hour insulins greater than 30 and less than 60 microunits per milliliter—supplemented by the third-hour measurements—identified hyperinsulinemia in all with second-hour values *greater than 40 microunits*, irrespective of the glucose tolerance status.

5) Irrespective of its value, whenever the second-hour insulin is the peak value—being greater than the one-hour value—hyperinsulinemia insulin Pattern III is identified. (See Chapter 12, Dynamic Insulin Patterns.)

Challenge #8

As many as 1 in 3 US adults could have diabetes by 2050 according to a new analysis from the Center for Disease Control and Prevention. This is not a surprise as so noted in Chapter 31. The publication titled *Projection for the year 2050 burden of diabetes in the US adult population: dynamic modeling of incidence, mortality and prediabetes prevalence* is in Population Health Metrics 22 October 2010. An electronic version can be found on line at http://www.pophealthmetrics.com/content/8/1/29.

The report projects the number of new cases of diabetes that will occur by 2050. Their projected costs of diabetes, judged opresive, are designated the national diabetes burden. Solutions to abort the diabetes epidemic were not proposed.

Until there is utilization of the very earliest diagnosis and treatment of type 1 and type 2 diabetes, i.e. the insulin assay with oral glucose tolerance, the estimates of 2050 will occur. Applying the insulin assay with oral glucose tolerance to ongoing national and international detection studies, especially of the young, is a practical application of screening for type 1 and type 2 diabetes. This screening will have a significant mitigating impact on the occurance of adult diabetes and its associated economic and human cost.

This book emphasizes that the Diabetes Epidemic can be reversed. The success of the earliest diagnosis and treatment will abort the world wide epidemic of diabetes which has impounded national and international medicine.

Challenge #9

What does YOUR future hold? This question is one that many of us do not want to address, at least not too often. The message of this book is that the diabetes epidemic affecting all age groups is a reality, and each one of us may be a part of it. The essence of the message is that you can do something about it. The choice is yours!

Challenge #10

Final Question:

SHOULD EVERYONE BE TESTED?

Final Answer:

ABSOLUTELY NOT!

ONLY THOSE CONCERNED ABOUT THEIR FUTURE!

Lightning Source UK Ltd.
Milton Keynes UK
UKHW011837111219
355187UK00001B/380/P